THE RENAL DIET MEAL PREP FOR THE NEWLY DIAGNOSED

Delicious Low-Sodium Potassium Recipes to Manage Kidney Disease

Adam C.

DEDICATION

This book is dedicated to all my Readers

CONTENTS

Chapter 1: Introduction

1.1 Understanding Kidney Disease

Millions of individuals throughout the world suffer with kidney disease, a quiet and sometimes misdiagnosed medical illness. Because they remove waste and extra fluid from the blood, balance electrolytes, and create hormones that lower blood pressure, the kidneys are essential for maintaining general health. These processes are hampered by kidney impairment, which causes the body to accumulate toxins and interferes with essential physiological functioning.

Chronic kidney disease (CKD) is a chronic illness that progresses over time and frequently has no symptoms at first. Numerous conditions, such as diabetes, hypertension, genetic predispositions, and specific drugs, can cause it. People may suffer from symptoms like anemia, weariness, edema, and changes in urine output as their kidney function deteriorates. Untreated chronic kidney disease (CKD) can lead to end-stage renal disease (ESRD), which makes dialysis or a kidney transplant necessary for survival.

Knowing the many stages of chronic kidney disease (CKD), identifying the risk factors, and taking preventive action are all important components of understanding kidney disease. Managing and reducing the course of this disorder requires regular blood tests to evaluate kidney function and adherence to a healthy lifestyle.

1.2 Importance of a Renal Diet

A key component of controlling renal disease and delaying its progression is diet. Key dietary components like salt, potassium, phosphorus, and protein are under strict control in a renal diet, which is especially designed to promote kidney function. These modifications assist in preserving a balance that promotes general health and lessen the strain on the kidneys.

Managing electrolyte and fluid imbalances is one of the main objectives of a renal diet. Sodium is a common ingredient in salt and is linked to high blood pressure and fluid retention, both of which can put stress on the kidneys. Potassium is an essential mineral that is needed for many different body processes, but too much of it can be dangerous for people whose kidney function is compromised.

Furthermore, since the breakdown of protein results in waste products that the kidneys must filter, it is imperative to keep an eye on the amount of protein consumed. Reducing phosphorus intake is also essential because excessive consumption can cause problems with the heart and bones.

Restrictions are just one aspect of adopting a renal diet; another is choosing scrumptious and nutritious foods that enhance general health. People can take an active role in managing their kidney health by being aware of the nutritional value of the foods they eat and choosing them carefully.

1.3 Benefits of Meal Preparation for Kidney Health

Meal preparation becomes a valuable tool in the management of kidney disease, especially for those who are newly diagnosed with renal diseases. Beyond just being convenient, meal preparation has a significant positive influence on nutrient intake, dietary adherence, and general health. Here are a few main benefits:

1. Portion Control: A key component of administering a renal diet is accurate portion control, which is made possible by meal preparation. People can limit their sodium intake, calorie intake, and consumption of other important nutrients by pre-measuring and portioning their meals.

2. Nutritional Awareness: Making meals at home and planning them help to improve nutritional awareness. This entails being aware of the nutritional value of different components, finding out about kidney-friendly substitutes, and making well-informed decisions that comply with dietary recommendations.

3. Customization: Dietary requirements vary from person to person. Preparing meals gives people the ability to tailor them to their tastes, health objectives, and unique renal needs. This adaptability guarantees long-lasting and pleasurable dietary changes.

4. Cost-Effective: Preparing meals at home is frequently less expensive than eating out or buying pre-packaged food. People can prioritize their health and manage their money by buying fresh products in bulk and making efficient use of them during meal preparation.

5. Time-Efficient: Despite popular belief, cooking healthfully doesn't have to take a lot of time. In the long term, meal preparation can save time. Batch cooking reduces the amount of time spent in the kitchen every day by enabling the preparation of several dishes at once.

6. Reduced Stress: The worry and anxiety brought on by dietary limitations can be lessened by knowing that kidney-friendly foods are easily accessible. Preparing meals gives one a sense of empowerment and control, which helps one maintain a positive outlook despite receiving a kidney diagnosis.

In-depth discussions of renal diet concepts, key components of kidney-friendly meals, and useful meal planning techniques will be covered in the upcoming chapters. People can start a journey to control kidney disease and enjoy exquisite flavors that contribute to a joyful and health-conscious existence by embracing the

benefits of meal preparation.

Chapter 2: Getting Started with the Renal Diet

It can be somewhat daunting to receive a new kidney disease diagnosis, but taking proactive measures to manage your health include learning about the principles of a renal diet and formulating a plan of action. This chapter will cover the key elements of beginning a renal diet, such as providing an overview of the guidelines, stressing the value of speaking with a healthcare provider, and emphasizing the need of establishing reasonable dietary objectives.

2.1 Overview of Renal Diet Guidelines

A renal diet limits the consumption of specific substances that can strain the kidneys in an effort to support kidney function. The main elements to concentrate on are as follows:

1. Sodium Control: An essential part of fluid balance is sodium, which is a key ingredient in table salt. On the other hand, consuming too much salt can cause fluid retention and high blood pressure, which can strain the kidneys. Restricting sodium consumption is generally advised by renal diet guidelines, which entail staying away from processed foods, eating out, and using too much salt when cooking.

Practical Tip: To cut back on salt usage and still have delectable meals, embrace the use of herbs, spices, and other flavor-enhancing substitutes.

2. Potassium Regulation: Although potassium is a necessary mineral for many body processes, such as heart and muscle function, people with renal illness may find it difficult to control their potassium levels. An excessive amount of potassium can be dangerous and cause problems including irregular heartbeats. Restricting high-potassium foods such bananas, oranges, tomatoes, and potatoes is often advised by renal diet guidelines.

Practical Tip: When consuming moderate-potassium meals, watch portion sizes and choose low-potassium options like apples, berries, and cauliflower.

3. Protein Moderation: Protein is essential for preserving muscle mass and promoting general health. But consuming too much protein can result in waste products that the kidneys have to filter.

Protein intake should be moderated while selecting high-quality sources, such as lean meats, poultry, fish, eggs, and plant-based proteins like tofu and lentils, according to renal diet guidelines.

Practical Tip: Consult a dietician to ascertain your individual protein requirements and space out your protein consumption throughout the day.

4. Phosphorus Management: Phosphorus, which is included in a variety of foods, can build up in the blood when kidney function is compromised, which can cause problems with the heart and bones. Most renal diet guidelines advise avoiding high-phosphorus foods like nuts, dairy, and some processed meals.

Practical Tip: Look into phosphorus binders as recommended by your healthcare provider, select lower-phosphorus options, and be aware of hidden phosphorus in packaged meals.

5. Fluid Balance: People with renal illness must maintain a proper fluid balance, particularly because their kidneys may find it difficult to control their fluid intake. Renal diet guidelines frequently contain suggestions for daily fluid intake that take into account individual parameters including exercise level, climate, and urine output.

Practical Tip: Track your fluid consumption and make necessary adjustments based on your level of exercise, thirst, and the advice of your healthcare team.

2.2 Consulting with a Healthcare Professional

It is not advisable to start a renal diet on your own. Getting advice from a medical professional is crucial for creating a customized and successful food plan, especially from a licensed dietitian or nutritionist with experience in kidney health.

1. The Role of a Registered Dietitian: A renal nutrition specialist registered dietitian can offer priceless advice on creating a well-balanced and pleasurable renal diet. They will evaluate your own health state, medical background, and nutritional preferences in order to design a personalized plan that meets your unique requirements.

Practical Tip: Request a referral to a licensed dietitian with knowledge in renal nutrition from your healthcare practitioner.

2. Collaboration with Your Healthcare Team: Working together with your healthcare team as a whole, not just dietitians, is essential. Your primary care physician, nephrologist, and any other specialists treating you may fall under this category. Your food plan will be in line with your overall treatment and health objectives if there is open communication.

Practical Tip: During routine check-ups, discuss your nutritional objectives and preferences with your healthcare team to get advice and modifications as needed.

3. Monitoring and Adjusting Medications: Dietary modifications may affect how well some drugs work. If you make any dietary changes, it's critical to let your healthcare provider know so that any required prescription adjustments can be done.

Practical Tip: Document any dietary modifications you make and present your doctor with a copy of it when you see them.

2.3 Setting Realistic Dietary Goals

Setting attainable dietary objectives is essential to long-term success when implementing a renal diet, which requires a substantial lifestyle modification. To create goals that are attainable, think about doing the following actions:

1. Gradual Changes: Try to make small, long-lasting modifications to your diet instead of trying to make a big, overnight overhaul. By taking this method, you can become accustomed to new eating habits and improve your chances of sticking with them over time.

Practical Tip: To begin, decide which one or two areas of your diet you can easily change. For example, you may cut back on sodium or increase the amount of snacks that are good for your kidneys.

2. Individualized Approach: Acknowledge that each person has different nutritional requirements and preferences. Create a strategy with your medical team that takes into account your lifestyle, cultural preferences, and individual health goals.

Practical Tip: Talk to your dietician about your preferred foods and cooking methods to identify kidney-friendly substitutes that you would like.

3. Regular Monitoring and Adjustments: A renal diet is dynamic and must be continuously evaluated and modified in accordance with your overall health, test findings, and state of health. Having routine check-ups with your healthcare team gives you the chance to assess your progress and make any necessary adjustments.

Practical Tip: Maintain a food journal to monitor your intake of meals, snacks, and liquids. When you visit with your nutritionist, share this information with them for tailored advice.

4. Celebrate Small Victories: Celebrate each little victory you achieve while following a renal diet. Any accomplishment, be it mastering a new kidney-friendly cuisine or routinely hitting your daily water intake targets, should be celebrated since it helps foster a good outlook.

Practical Tip: To boost motivation and a sense of achievement, set short-term goals and treat yourself when you reach them.

To sum up, in order to begin a renal diet, one must comprehend the basic rules, consult a healthcare provider, and establish reasonable dietary objectives. Those who have just received a kidney disease diagnosis can establish a long-term, health-conscious management strategy for their illness by adopting these guidelines. The practical features of meal planning, necessary ingredients and mouthwatering recipes that make the renal diet not only doable but pleasurable will be covered in more detail in the upcoming chapters.

Chapter 3: Essential Ingredients for Renal-Friendly Meal Prep

A renal diet journey includes adopting a range of foods that promote kidney health in addition to avoiding specific items. We will examine the necessary components for renal-friendly meal preparation in this chapter, emphasizing low-sodium alternatives, potassium-controlled items, premium protein sources, and the inclusion of healthy fats.

3.1 Low-Sodium Options

A key component of the renal diet is cutting back on salt since too much of it can cause fluid retention and high blood pressure, which further tax the kidneys. You can enhance the flavor of your meals without jeopardizing the health of your kidneys by adopting low-sodium solutions.

1. Herbs and Spices: If you want to add more flavor to your food without using salt, herbs and spices work great. Try experimenting with other herbs and spices, including cumin, turmeric, and garlic powder, and herbs like basil, thyme, rosemary, and cilantro.

Practical Tip: To give your recipes more depth and complexity, make your own herb mixes. For an Italian-inspired spice, combine garlic, basil, and oregano.

2. Vinegars with Citrus: Balsamic and apple cider vinegars in particular can give your food sour and acidic undertones. Lemons and limes are examples of citrus fruits that bring brightness without using a lot of salt.

Practical Tip: To add a flavorful burst to cooked dishes, squeeze fresh citrus juice over them and use vinegar-based dressings for salads and marinades.

3. Low-Sodium Condiments: Look into alternatives to common condiments like hot sauce, Worcestershire sauce, and soy sauce that are lower in salt. You may follow the recommendations for the renal diet and still enjoy the comforting flavors with these substitutes.

Practical Tip: Look for condiments branded "low-sodium" or "sodium-free" and check the labels for the sodium content.

4. Homemade Stocks and Broths: While store-bought stocks and broths may contain a lot of sodium, making your own gives you more control over the amount of salt. Make tasty, low-sodium soup and stew bases with lean meats, fresh veggies, and herbs.

Practical Tip: Make large batches of homemade broth and freeze in smaller portions for convenient use in various recipes.

5. Fresh and Frozen Vegetables: In their unprocessed state, vegetables are rich in important nutrients and low in salt. Try to avoid adding salt to your fresh or frozen veggies, and try different cooking techniques to bring out the tastes.

Practical Tip: You can enhance the flavor of veggies without adding too much salt by roasting, grilling, or sautéing them with herbs and spices.

3.2 Potassium-Controlled Ingredients

For those with renal illness, maintaining a balanced potassium intake is essential since compromised kidneys may find it difficult to control potassium levels. Although you should limit some high-potassium items, your renal diet can still be varied with lots of tasty choices.

1. Low-Potassium Fruits: Include fruits including apples, berries, grapes, and peaches that have a reduced potassium level. These choices offer natural sweetness without putting you at risk of consuming too much potassium.

Practical Tip: For a cool and kidney-friendly treat, try varying the fruit combinations in salads, smoothies, and desserts.

2. Lower-Potassium Vegetables: Select veggies such as cucumber, bell peppers, zucchini, and cauliflower that are lower in potassium. These choices enhance your meals with color, texture, and nutrients without raising your potassium levels.

Practical Tip: Mix various low-potassium veggies with fresh herbs and a squeeze of lemon to create colorful and interesting salads.

3. Soaking and Boiling Techniques: You can lower the potassium content of some high-potassium foods by soaking and boiling them. For instance, you can soak and boil potatoes and beans to extract extra potassium.

Practical Tip: To properly control potassium levels, soak dried beans and boil potatoes before adding them to your dishes.

4. Portion Control: It's important to exercise portion control even though you may still include some foods with greater potassium in your diet. You can manage your potassium consumption and yet enjoy a variety of foods when you practice moderation.

Practical Tip: Use smaller portions of higher-potassium ingredients in mixed dishes, balancing them with lower-potassium options.

5. Consultation with a Dietitian: Consult your dietician frequently to customize your potassium intake to meet your individual requirements. They can help you select the appropriate fruits, vegetables, and other items based on your dietary objectives and unique health situation.

Practical Tip: Make regular visits to talk about your potassium levels and to discuss any changes that should be made to your food plan with your dietitian.

3.3 Choosing High-Quality Protein Sources

A healthy diet must include protein since it promotes general health and muscle growth. But, people with renal illness must watch how much protein they eat and select high-quality sources that support good nutrition without taxing the kidneys too much.

1. Lean Meats: Choose lean meats such turkey, pig loin, and skinless chicken. Before cooking, trim any visible fats to lower your consumption of saturated fat, which is good for your heart.

Practical Tip: To enhance the flavor of lean meats without using too much salt, try experimenting with different marinades and rubs.

2. Fish and Seafood: These foods are great providers of premium protein. Omega-3 fatty acids, which promote heart health, are found in fatty seafood like salmon and mackerel.

Practical Tip: For a tasty and kidney-friendly main course, bake, broil, or grill fish with citrus and herbs.

3. Plant-Based Proteins: Include sources of plant-based protein include beans, tofu, and tempeh. In addition to protein, these substitutes also include fiber and a variety of vitamins and minerals.

Practical Tip: Try a variety of recipes, including as bean salads and tofu stir-fries that highlight the adaptability of plant-based proteins.

4. Eggs and Egg Whites: While utilizing egg whites can lower phosphorus intake while preserving protein levels, eggs are still a great source of protein. Add eggs to your meals boiled, scrambled, or added to casseroles.

Practical Tip: For a wholesome and filling breakfast or lunch, make an omelet with egg whites, veggies, and herbs that is kidney-friendly.

5. Dairy Substitutes: If phosphorus limitations force you to restrict your dairy intake, take into account dairy substitutes such almond, rice, or oat milk. To assist bone health, these alternatives can be fortified with calcium and vitamin D.

Practical Tip: Find your favorite non-dairy milk by

experimenting and using dairy substitutes in cereals, coffee, and smoothies.

3.4 Incorporating Healthy Fats

Incorporating healthy fats is just as important as controlling sodium, potassium, and protein in a renal diet. Fats contribute to flavor, satiety, and the absorption of nutrients. Making heart-healthy fat choices promotes cardiovascular health, which is crucial for those with renal disease.

1. Olive Oil: Olive oil is a heart-healthy fat that adds richness to dishes. Use it for sautéing, roasting, or drizzling over salads to enhance flavors without relying on excessive salt.

Practical Tip: Experiment with different varieties of olive oil, such as extra virgin or infused options, to discover new dimensions of taste.

2. Avocado: Avocado is a nutrient-dense fruit that provides healthy monounsaturated fats. Mash it for spreads, slices for salads, or blend into smoothies for creaminess.

Practical Tip: Create a kidney-friendly guacamole with diced tomatoes, onions, cilantro, and lime juice for a flavorful dip.

3. Nuts and Seeds: Nuts and seeds are excellent sources of healthy fats, fiber, and essential nutrients. Choose unsalted varieties to manage sodium intake and enjoy them as snacks or sprinkled over salads and yogurt.

Practical Tip: Roast nuts and seeds with your favorite herbs and spices for a tasty and kidney-friendly snack.

4. Fatty Fish: Add omega-3 fatty acids to your diet by including fatty fish like trout, salmon, and mackerel. These heart-healthy fats enhance the flavor of your food and support cardiovascular health.

Practical Tip: For a tasty and kidney-friendly main meal, marinate fatty fish in a marinade of lemon and herbs and grill or bake.

5. Coconut Products: You can add taste by using coconut goods in moderation, such as coconut oil, coconut milk, and coconut shreds. Even though they are heavy in saturated fat, they may give your recipes a tropical flavor when used judiciously.

Practical Tip: Try different curries made with coconut milk or top kidney-friendly sweets with shredded coconut.

Including these key items in your renal-friendly meal prep offers up a world of tasty and fulfilling culinary possibilities in addition to supporting kidney health. You'll find that a renal diet may be tasty and fulfilling as you try out various flavors and combinations. You will learn how to prepare delicious and successful renal-friendly meals by following the chapters that follow, which include recipes and helpful meal planning advice.

Chapter 4: Weekly Meal Planning for Kidney Health

The key to handling a renal diet successfully is meal planning. This chapter will walk you through creating balanced meals, offer advice on controlling portion sizes, and provide you ideas on how to modify well-known recipes to make them renal-friendly. You may maintain a delicious and kidney-conscious diet that promotes your overall health with careful planning and inventive modifications.

4.1 Building Balanced Meals

Planning meals that are both nutritionally adequate and compliant with renal diet standards is crucial. A diverse range of nutrient-dense meals that support general health are included on a well-rounded plate. Now let's examine the components of creating meals that are balanced for renal health:

1. Include a Variety of Vegetables: Packed with vitamins, minerals, and antioxidants, vegetables are an essential component of a diet that is beneficial to the kidneys. Try to load up half of your plate with a rainbow of vibrant non-starchy veggies, such broccoli, cauliflower, bell peppers, and leafy greens.

Practical Tip: To improve the flavors and textures of your vegetables, try experimenting with different cooking techniques like roasting, grilling, or sautéing.

2. Choose Lean Protein Sources: Include lean protein sources to maintain the health of your muscles without overtaxing your kidneys. Lean meats, fish, eggs, skinless chicken and plant-based proteins like tofu or lentils are your best options.

Practical Tip: To guarantee a consistent supply of amino acids without unduly taxing your kidneys, spread out the amount of protein you eat throughout the day.

3. Include Whole Grains: Whole grains offer fiber, vital nutrients, and long-lasting energy. To enhance your meals, select whole grains like barley, quinoa, brown rice, and whole wheat products.

Practical Tip: To add diversity to your diet, try experimenting with different grains. For a novel twist, try adding ancient grains like freekeh or farro.

4. Monitor Potassium Intake: Choose fruits and vegetables that are lower in potassium to be conscious of how much you eat. Balance is maintained by offering a range of options and practicing moderation.

Practical Tip: To maintain diversity and properly control potassium levels, alternate between low- and moderate-potassium alternatives.

5. Limit Phosphorus-Rich Foods: Be mindful of your phosphorus intake in addition to your potassium intake. To maintain kidney health, limit high-phosphorus foods such dairy products, nuts, and some processed foods.

Practical Tip: Look into phosphorus binders and choose dairy substitutes with reduced phosphorus content, as advised by your medical staff.

6. Incorporate Healthy Fats: Use foods like almonds, avocados, olive oil, and fatty seafood to provide heart-healthy fats to your meals. These fats enhance general health and give your food a delightful taste.

Practical Tip: To improve the flavor of your food, use tiny amounts of healthy fats in dressings, toppings, and cooking.

7. Watch Sodium Intake: Reduce your intake of sodium by utilizing herbs, spices, and other flavor-enhancing ingredients along with low-sodium substitutes. Salt reduction supports renal function and helps manage fluid retention.

Practical Tip: Use more herbs, spices, and other flavors free of sodium while gradually reducing your intake of salt.

4.2 Tips for Portion Control

In order to maintain a healthy weight, monitor nutrient levels, and manage calorie consumption, portion control is essential when following a renal diet. The following are some useful pointers for efficient portion control:

1. Use Smaller Plates: To provide the impression of a fuller plate with fewer pieces, use smaller plates. You may control serving sizes with this visual trick without feeling cheated.

Practical Tip: To promote proper portion proportions, select 8–

9-inch-diameter plates for main meals.

2. Measure Portions: To precisely measure ingredients and servings, use scales, measuring cups, and other portion control instruments. By doing this, you can be sure that you are conscious of your intake and can modify it as necessary.

Practical Tip: Gradually move from measuring portions to guessing based on visual cues as you gain an understanding of proper serving proportions.

3. Listen to Hunger and Fullness Cues: Observe the cues your body gives you about hunger and fullness. By taking your time and enjoying every meal, you can identify when you're full and avoid overindulging.

Practical Tip: Take a moment during your meal to gauge your appetite. Choose to eat extra servings of non-starchy vegetables if you're still hungry.

4. Dividing Your Plate: Imagine your plate to be divided into three sections: one quarter for whole grains, one quarter for lean protein, and one half for non-starchy veggies. This methodology guarantees an equitable dispersion of nutrients.

Practical Tip: To guarantee a well-balanced and kidney-friendly composition, using the plate dividing method as a reference when serving meals.

5. Pre-Portion Snacks: Before indulging in snacks, divide them into individual baggies or tiny containers. This keeps you from overindulging and improves your ability to regulate portion sizes.

Practical Tip: For easy and regulated snacking, prepare snack-sized servings of fruits, almonds, or whole-grain crackers ahead of time.

6. Share Larger Portions: If you're cooking or eating out, think about splitting larger servings with a friend or relative. This enables you to savor a range of flavors without going overboard with the amount you eat.

Practical Tip: For individual meals, divide larger dishes into smaller quantities or opt to split an entrée at a restaurant.

7. Be Mindful of Liquid Calories: Soups and beverages might contain calories that should be taken into consideration. Choose low-sodium broths, herbal teas, and water to stay hydrated without consuming too many calories.

Practical Tip: To improve awareness of your drink consumption, use smaller glasses and enjoy every sip.

4.3 Adapting Familiar Recipes to Renal-Friendly Versions

Renal diet compatibility allows you to prioritize kidney health while still enjoying your favorite cuisines by modifying well-known recipes. Here's how to change recipes without compromising flavor:

1. Modify Cooking Methods: Try a variety of cooking techniques to cut back on the amount of salt you use. Natural tastes can be enhanced by grilling, roasting, baking, steaming, and sautéing without going against the rules of the renal diet.

Practical Tip: For a tasty and kidney-friendly side dish, grill veggies with a splash of olive oil and a sprinkling of herbs.

2. Reduce Salt Gradually: Give your taste buds time to adjust by gradually cutting back on the amount of salt in your dishes. Your sensitivity to salt will gradually lessen, and you'll come to value the flavors that items naturally have.

Practical Tip: As your taste buds adjust, start by halving the quantity of salt you use and then progressively reduce it from there.

3. Explore salt-Free Seasonings: Use seasonings like herbs, spices, garlic, onion, and lemon juice in place of salt. These substitutions give your meals more depth and complexity without increasing your sodium intake.

Practical Tip: Make your own seasoning blends without added salt to use in soups and marinades, among other recipes.

4. Choose Low-Sodium Ingredients: Whenever possible, choose low-sodium versions of ingredients. This covers processed foods, canned goods, broths, and condiments. Choosing goods with lower sodium content and reading labels can help you control how much salt you eat overall.

Practical Tip: When making renal-friendly meal preparations, compare product labels and select those with the lowest sodium level.

5. Limit High-Potassium Ingredients: Replace ingredients with Lower Potassium in recipes calling for high-potassium components. To preserve color and flavor without raising potassium levels, swap out tomatoes in a recipe with bell peppers.

Practical Tip: Find appropriate replacements for high-potassium components in your favorite dishes by consulting with your nutritionist.

6. Experiment with Phosphorus Binders: If your diet calls for stringent phosphorus management, consider using phosphorus binders as advised by your medical professionals. These drugs may be able to counteract the absorption of phosphorus, giving you greater options when it comes to recipes.

Practical Advice: To include phosphorus binder choices and usage into your renal diet, talk to your healthcare professional.

7. Portion Control in Casseroles: Be mindful of the amount of high-potassium or high-phosphorus components you use in casseroles and one-pot meals. By evenly distributing these ingredients throughout the dish, moderation is ensured without compromising flavor.

Practical Tip: Make sure you use a range of kidney-friendly substitutes and use fewer amounts of high-potassium items.

You can effectively navigate a kidney-conscious diet without sacrificing flavor or enjoyment by creating balanced meals, exercising portion control, and modifying well-known recipes to renal-friendly alternatives. The following chapters will go over certain meal plans and recipes that will help your renal diet experience be both pleasurable and doable. Continuing to discover the delectable potential of preparing renal-friendly meals will reveal that looking after your kidneys can be a satisfying and tasty endeavor.

Chapter 5: Renal Diet Meal Prep Tools and Techniques

An effective way to prepare meals is essential to following a renal diet. The use of meal prep containers, batch cooking techniques, and advice on storing and reheating kidney-friendly meals are just a few of the crucial tools and methods we'll cover in this chapter to help you prepare meals faster for the renal diet.

5.1 Meal Prep Containers

A vital first step in making sure your renal-friendly meals are practical, well-organized, and manageable is selecting the appropriate meal prep containers. When picking out meal prep containers, take into account the following factors:

1. Size and Portion Control: To help with portion management, choose containers made for single servings. In particular, divided containers with distinct sections for grains, vegetables, and proteins are useful for preparing meals that are well-balanced.

Practical Tip: Purchase containers in different sizes so that you can customize meal components and portion amounts according to your dietary requirements.

2. Freezer-Safe and Microwaveable: To preserve the quality of your food while storing and reheating, select containers that are both freezer-safe and microwave-safe. This adaptability makes it easy to go from preparing meals to indulging in kidney-friendly cuisine.

Practical Tip: Seek for packaging made for frequent freezing and microwaving that is labeled as BPA-free.

3. Airtight Seals: To maintain the freshness of your meals and avoid freezer burn, make sure that the meal prep containers have tight, airtight seals. In the refrigerator, airtight containers also aid in flavor retention and help avoid cross-contamination.

Practical Tip: To prevent leaks and preserve the best possible food quality, test the seals on your containers before freezing meals.

4. Stackable Design: To optimize storage space in your freezer or refrigerator, select containers with a stackable design. Multiple meals can be easily arranged and accessed with stackable containers, which save a lot of shelf space.

Practical Tip: Label and access individual meals with ease by arranging containers in an orderly fashion when needed.

5. Reusable and Eco-Friendly: When preparing meals, use reusable containers to cut waste and encourage sustainability. Seek for containers with materials that are strong enough to endure repeated use without losing their integrity.

Practical Tip: To keep your containers in good shape for extended usage, wash and sterilize them on a regular basis.

5.2 Batch Cooking Strategies

Making several portions of a dish at once is known as batch cooking, and it's an effective and time-saving method that lets you enjoy fresh meals on a less frequent basis. Using batch cooking in conjunction with your renal diet can streamline your preparation process and offer a range of kidney-friendly choices.

1. Choose Versatile Recipes: Choose recipes that are flexible enough to be modified for different dinners during the week. Recipes that may be portioned and consumed over many days, such as casseroles, stews, and soups, work well when prepared in batches.

Practical Tip: To add variation to your batch-cooked dishes, try experimenting with different spice blends and seasonings.

2. Invest in Quality Storage Containers: Make an investment in storage containers of the highest caliber that may be used to freeze and chill meals prepared in bulk. Servings of your food will always be as tasty thanks to the use of proper containers, which help maintain the flavors and textures of your food.

Practical Tip: Write the date of preparation on containers to keep track of freshness and help you choose meals that are well-informed.

3. Portion and Label before Freezing: Before freezing, divide up your batch-cooked meals into individual portions. This lowers the possibility of thawing and reheating more food than is required by making it simple to grab a single meal when needed.

Practical Tip: For easy reference, label containers with the dish's name, the preparation date, and any reheating instructions.

4. Rotate and Plan Variety: To guarantee that you have a wide range of meals to pick from throughout the week, schedule your batch cooking sessions to incorporate a variety of dishes. For a renal diet that is both balanced and pleasurable, switch up your protein, grain, and vegetable intake.

Practical Tip: Based on your dietary choices and nutritional needs, make a weekly meal plan to help you organize your batch cooking sessions.

5. Time-Saving Ingredients: Select items that make batch cooking easier, to cut down on preparation time without sacrificing the nutritious value of your meals, try utilizing pre-cut vegetables, canned beans, or pre-cooked grains.

Practical Tip: To make choosing ingredients for batch cooking easier, stock your freezer and cupboard with kidney-friendly essentials.

5.3 Freezing and Reheating Tips

Meal prep and freezing are essential for maintaining the safety and quality of your renal-friendly recipes. To guarantee that the taste and nutritional content of your frozen meals are maintained, adhere to following guidelines:

1. Cool Meals before Freezing: Before freezing prepared meals, let them cool to room temperature. Quick chilling preserves the texture of the components and stops ice crystals from forming, which can degrade the quality of frozen food.

Practical Tip: To expedite the cooling process, divide large batches into smaller parts.

2. Use Freezer-Safe Packaging: To avoid freezer burn and preserve the freshness of your food, choose freezer-safe packaging. Refrigerator-safe bags, airtight jars, and sturdy aluminum foil are good choices for freezing kidney-friendly recipes.

Practical Tip: To reduce the chance of freezer burn, take out as much air as you can from freezer bags or containers.

3. Label Containers Clearly: Make sure that the name of the dish, the preparation date, and any reheating instructions are clearly labeled on every frozen meal. By using this information, you can make sure that you eat meals within the best possible storage period and stay on top of what's in your freezer.

Realistic Tip: Establish a labeling scheme that makes it simple to identify and switch out frozen meals.

4. Reheat with Care: When reheating frozen food, take care to maintain the texture and flavor of the food. Depending on the food, there are typical choices such as microwaving, stovetop reheating, and oven baking.

Practical Tip: To avoid dryness and improve overall dish wetness, add a dash of broth or water during reheating.

5. Avoid Overcooking: Pay attention to when to reheat meals to prevent overcooking frozen food. Flavor loss and dryness can arise from overcooking. Reheat food according to the suggested timings, and occasionally make sure it's done.

Practical Tip: To guarantee even heating throughout, stir frozen casseroles or stews every few minutes while they are being reheated.

6. Thaw Safely: To reduce the chance of bacterial growth, defrost frozen meals in a safe manner. Meals can be thawed in the fridge, in a sealed plastic bag submerged in cold water, or by utilizing the defrost feature on a microwave.

Practical Tip: Schedule your meals in advance, especially for larger dishes, to give yourself enough time to safely thaw them in the refrigerator.

7. Reheat Soups and Stews Gradually: To prevent overheating and possible nutrient loss, slowly reheat soups and stews. To ensure that heat is distributed evenly, start with a lower heat setting and increase as necessary, stirring from time to time.

Practical Tip: To bring back flavors and intensify aromas in your soups, add freshly chopped herbs or a splash of lemon juice after reheating.

You may make your meal prep for the renal diet effective, structured, and sustainable by using meal prep containers, using batch cooking techniques, and adhering to freezing and reheating guidelines. With the help of these methods and instruments, you may continue to prepare a range of kidney-friendly dishes, giving you flexibility and convenience in your everyday cooking activities. You'll experience the convenience and satisfaction of supporting your kidney health journey with wholesome, cooked meals always on hand as you incorporate these practices into your daily routine.

Chapter 6: Breakfast Recipes

A hearty breakfast establishes the framework for the rest of the day and supplies vital nutrients to maintain your general health while following the recommendations of a renal diet. This chapter will include three delectable kidney-friendly breakfast recipes: Whole Grain Pancakes with Fruit Compote, Egg White and Vegetable Frittata, and Low-Sodium Oatmeal with Berries.

6.1 Low-Sodium Oatmeal with Berries

A simple way to make oatmeal fit the needs of a renal diet is to make it more heart-healthy and adaptable. You may make a tasty and kidney-friendly breakfast by adding fresh berries and selecting low-sodium toppings.

Ingredients:

- 1/2 cup old-fashioned oats
- 1 cup water
- 1/2 cup fresh berries (such as blueberries, strawberries, or raspberries)
- 1 tablespoon chopped nuts (almonds or walnuts), optional
- 1 teaspoon honey or maple syrup, optional

- Cinnamon, to taste

- Low-sodium milk or dairy-free alternative, to serve

Instructions:

1. In a saucepan, bring 1 cup of water to a boil.

2. Stir in the old-fashioned oats and reduce the heat to a simmer. Cook the oats according to the package instructions, usually for about 5-7 minutes, stirring occasionally.

3. Once the oats are cooked, remove the saucepan from heat and let it sit for a minute to thicken.

4. Transfer the oatmeal to a bowl and top it with fresh berries.

5. Sprinkle chopped nuts, if using, over the berries for added texture and flavor.

6. Drizzle honey or maple syrup over the oats for a touch of sweetness, if desired.

7. Finish with a sprinkle of cinnamon to enhance the overall flavor.

8. Serve the low-sodium oatmeal with a splash of low-sodium milk or a dairy-free alternative of your choice.

Practical Tip: Experiment with different combinations of berries and nuts to discover your favorite flavor profile. Adjust the sweetness level according to your taste preferences, and enjoy a satisfying and kidney-friendly breakfast that provides a good source of fiber and antioxidants.

6.2 Egg White and Vegetable Frittata

Eggs are a protein-rich breakfast option, and by using egg whites and incorporating a variety of colorful vegetables, you can create a flavorful and kidney-friendly frittata. This recipe offers a delicious way to start your day with a boost of protein and essential nutrients.

Ingredients:

- 6 egg whites
- 1/4 cup diced bell peppers (assorted colors)
- 1/4 cup diced tomatoes
- 1/4 cup chopped spinach or kale
- 1/4 cup diced zucchini
- 1/4 cup diced red onion
- 1 tablespoon olive oil
- Salt and pepper, to taste
- Fresh herbs (such as parsley or chives), for garnish

Instructions:

1. Preheat the oven to 375°F (190°C).

2. In a mixing bowl, whisk the egg whites until frothy. Season with salt and pepper to taste.

3. Heat olive oil in an oven-safe skillet over medium heat.

4. Add diced bell peppers, tomatoes, spinach or kale, zucchini, and red onion to the skillet. Sauté the vegetables until they are slightly softened, about 3-5 minutes.

5. Pour the whisked egg whites over the sautéed vegetables, ensuring an even distribution.

6. Cook on the stovetop for 2-3 minutes, allowing the edges to set.

7. Transfer the skillet to the preheated oven and bake for 12-15 minutes or until the frittata is fully set and lightly browned on top.

8. Carefully remove the skillet from the oven and let the frittata cool slightly.

9. Garnish with fresh herbs, slice, and serve.

Practical Tip: Feel free to customize the frittata with your favorite vegetables or herbs. You can add low-potassium options like mushrooms, asparagus, or green beans to create a variety of delicious combinations. The frittata can be sliced and stored for quick and convenient breakfasts throughout the week.

6.3 Whole Grain Pancakes with Fruit Compote

Enjoying pancakes on a renal diet is possible by opting for whole grain variations and creating flavorful fruit compote without added sugars. This recipe provides a wholesome and satisfying breakfast option that aligns with kidney-friendly guidelines.

Ingredients:

For Pancakes:

- 1 cup whole wheat flour
- 1 tablespoon baking powder
- 1/2 teaspoon cinnamon
- 1 cup low-sodium milk or dairy-free alternative
- 1 large egg
- 1 tablespoon olive oil
- 1 teaspoon vanilla extract
- Fresh berries, for topping

For Fruit Compote:

- 1 cup mixed berries (such as strawberries, blueberries, and raspberries)
- 1 tablespoon water
- 1 teaspoon lemon juice

- 1 tablespoon honey or maple syrup, optional

Instructions:

For Pancakes:

1. In a mixing bowl, whisk together whole wheat flour, baking powder, and cinnamon.
2. In a separate bowl, whisk together low-sodium milk, egg, olive oil, and vanilla extract.
3. Pour the wet ingredients into the dry ingredients and stir until just combined. Let the batter rest for a few minutes.
4. Heat a griddle or non-stick skillet over medium heat. Lightly coat with cooking spray or a small amount of olive oil.
5. Pour 1/4 cup of batter onto the griddle for each pancake. Cook until bubbles form on the surface, then flip and cook the other side until golden brown.
6. Repeat until all the batter is used.

For Fruit Compote:

1. In a small saucepan, combine mixed berries, water, and lemon juice.
2. Cook over medium heat, stirring occasionally, until the berries break down and the mixture thickens, about 5-7 minutes.

3. If desired, sweeten the compote with honey or maple syrup. Adjust sweetness according to taste.

4. Remove the compote from heat and let it cool slightly.

To Serve:

- Stack the whole grain pancakes on a plate.
- Top with the mixed berry compote and fresh berries.
- Drizzle with additional honey or maple syrup, if desired.

Practical Tip: Experiment with different whole grains, such as oat flour or buckwheat flour, to add variety to your pancake recipe. The fruit compote can be prepared in advance and refrigerated, making it a convenient and kidney-friendly topping for your whole grain pancakes.

These breakfast recipes follow the guidelines of a renal diet but offer a delicious variety of flavors and textures. You may start your day on a delicious and kidney-friendly note by focusing on full, nutrient-dense foods and combining fresh, low-sodium components. Please feel free to modify these dishes to your own tastes and discover the many delicious options available for a renal-conscious breakfast.

Chapter 7: Lunch Ideas for Kidney Health

Lunch is an important meal that you should eat every day. You may make tasty, filling meals that promote your overall health by focusing on kidney-friendly items. This chapter will discuss three delectable lunch options that adhere to the strictures of a renal diet: Quinoa and Black Bean Bowl; Turkey and Avocado Wrap with Renal-Friendly Spread; Grilled Chicken Salad with Fresh Vegetables.

7.1 Grilled Chicken Salad with Fresh Vegetables

A refreshing and nutrient-packed salad is an excellent choice for a kidney-friendly lunch. By incorporating grilled chicken and a variety of fresh vegetables, you can create a vibrant and satisfying dish that is both delicious and supportive of kidney health.

Ingredients:

For the Grilled Chicken:

- 1 boneless, skinless chicken breast
- 1 tablespoon olive oil
- 1 teaspoon dried oregano

- Salt and pepper, to taste

For the Salad:

- Mixed salad greens (lettuce, spinach, arugula, or a combination)
- Cherry tomatoes, halved
- Cucumber, sliced
- Red bell pepper, sliced
- Red onion, thinly sliced
- Feta cheese, crumbled (optional)

For the Dressing:

- 2 tablespoons olive oil
- 1 tablespoon balsamic vinegar
- 1 teaspoon Dijon mustard
- 1 teaspoon honey
- Salt and pepper, to taste

Instructions:

For the Grilled Chicken:

1. Preheat the grill or grill pan over medium-high heat.
2. In a small bowl, mix olive oil, dried oregano, salt, and pepper to create a marinade.

3. Brush the marinade over the chicken breast, ensuring it is evenly coated.

4. Grill the chicken for 6-8 minutes per side or until fully cooked. Allow it to rest for a few minutes before slicing.

For the Salad:

1. In a large bowl, combine mixed salad greens, cherry tomatoes, cucumber, red bell pepper, and red onion.

2. Add the sliced grilled chicken on top of the salad.

3. If desired, sprinkle crumbled feta cheese over the salad for added flavor.

For the Dressing:

1. In a small bowl, whisk together olive oil, balsamic vinegar, Dijon mustard, honey, salt, and pepper until well combined.

2. Drizzle the dressing over the salad just before serving and toss gently to coat.

Practical Tip: Feel free to customize the salad by adding kidney-friendly vegetables like radishes, carrots, or green beans. Adjust the dressing ingredients according to your taste preferences, and enjoy a nutrient-rich and satisfying grilled chicken salad that supports your kidney health.

7.2 Quinoa and Black Bean Bowl

Quinoa is a protein-rich grain that serves as an excellent base for a kidney-friendly lunch bowl. By combining it with black beans and an assortment of colorful vegetables, you can create a well-balanced and flavorful meal that aligns with renal diet guidelines.

Ingredients:

- 1 cup cooked quinoa
- 1/2 cup canned black beans, rinsed and drained
- 1/2 cup corn kernels (fresh, frozen, or canned)
- 1/2 cup cherry tomatoes, halved
- 1/4 cup red onion, finely chopped
- 1/4 cup fresh cilantro, chopped
- 1 avocado, diced
- Lime wedges, for garnish

For the Dressing:

- 2 tablespoons olive oil
- 1 tablespoon lime juice
- 1 teaspoon ground cumin
- Salt and pepper, to taste

Instructions:

1. In a large bowl, combine cooked quinoa, black beans, corn kernels, cherry tomatoes, red onion, and cilantro.
2. In a small bowl, whisk together olive oil, lime juice, ground cumin, salt, and pepper to create the dressing.
3. Pour the dressing over the quinoa mixture and toss gently to coat.
4. Gently fold in diced avocado.
5. Serve the quinoa and black bean bowl in individual portions, garnished with lime wedges.

Practical Tip: Experiment with different herbs and spices to enhance the flavor profile of your quinoa and black bean bowl. You can add a touch of chili powder, paprika, or fresh parsley for additional depth. This versatile lunch option is not only delicious but also provides a good balance of protein, fiber, and essential nutrients.

7.3 Turkey and Avocado Wrap with Renal-Friendly Spread

A wrap is a convenient and portable lunch option, and by using lean turkey, creamy avocado, and a renal-friendly spread, you can create a satisfying and kidney-conscious meal that caters to your dietary needs.

Ingredients:

- 1 whole-grain or low-sodium tortilla

- 3 ounces lean turkey slices

- 1/2 avocado, sliced

- 1/4 cup shredded lettuce

- 1/4 cup cucumber, julienned

- 1 tablespoon renal-friendly spread (see recipe below)

Renal-Friendly Spread:

- 1/4 cup Greek yogurt (low-potassium)

- 1 teaspoon Dijon mustard

- 1 teaspoon lemon juice

- 1 teaspoon fresh dill, chopped

- Salt and pepper, to taste

Instructions:

For the Renal-Friendly Spread:

1. In a small bowl, mix together Greek yogurt, Dijon mustard, lemon juice, chopped fresh dill, salt, and pepper.
2. Adjust the seasoning according to taste and set aside.

For the Turkey and Avocado Wrap:

1. Lay the tortilla on a clean surface or a large plate.
2. Spread the renal-friendly spread evenly over the tortilla, leaving a small border around the edges.
3. Place the lean turkey slices on one side of the tortilla.
4. Arrange sliced avocado, shredded lettuce, and julienned cucumber on top of the turkey.
5. Fold in the sides of the tortilla and then roll it up tightly from the bottom to create a wrap.
6. Slice the wrap in half diagonally for easier handling.

Practical Tip: Feel free to customize the wrap with additional kidney-friendly vegetables, such as bell peppers or radishes. Adjust the thickness of the spread according to your preference, and enjoy a satisfying and portable lunch option that meets the dietary requirements of a renal-conscious meal.

These lunch ideas follow the guidelines of a renal diet yet offer a variety of tastes and textures. You can have tasty and healthy meals that promote kidney health by focusing on lean proteins, whole grains, and kidney-friendly spreads, and by combining fresh, low-sodium products. To make your trip with a renal diet enjoyable and long-lasting, think about tailoring these recipes to your nutritional requirements and personal taste preferences as

you try them out.

Chapter 8: Dinner Delights

Dinner is a chance to enjoy a substantial and fulfilling meal while following the guidelines of a renal diet. We will look at three delectable, kidney-friendly supper recipes in this chapter: Lentil and vegetable stew; stir-fried vegetables with tofu; baked salmon with lemon and herbs.

8.1 Baked Salmon with Lemon and Herbs

Salmon is a nutrient-rich fish that provides an excellent source of omega-3 fatty acids and high-quality protein. Baking salmon with fresh lemon and herbs creates a flavorful and heart-healthy dinner option that aligns with renal diet guidelines.

Ingredients:

- 2 salmon fillets
- 1 tablespoon olive oil
- 1 lemon, thinly sliced
- 2 tablespoons fresh dill, chopped
- 1 teaspoon dried oregano
- Salt and pepper, to taste

Instructions:

1. Preheat the oven to 375°F (190°C).
2. Place the salmon fillets on a baking sheet lined with parchment paper.
3. Drizzle olive oil over the salmon fillets, ensuring they are evenly coated.
4. Season the salmon with salt, pepper, and dried oregano.
5. Arrange lemon slices on top of each salmon fillet, and sprinkle fresh dill over the lemon slices.
6. Bake in the preheated oven for 15-20 minutes or until the salmon is cooked through and easily flakes with a fork.
7. Remove from the oven and let it rest for a few minutes before serving.

Practical Tip: Serve the baked salmon with a side of steamed low-potassium vegetables, such as green beans or asparagus, for a well-rounded and kidney-friendly dinner. Adjust the seasoning and herb choices based on your taste preferences, and enjoy a delicious and nutritious meal that supports kidney health.

8.2 Vegetable Stir-Fry with Tofu

A colorful and flavorful vegetable stir-fry with tofu provides a satisfying plant-based dinner option that is rich in vitamins, minerals, and protein. By incorporating a variety of kidney-friendly vegetables, you can create a delicious stir-fry that aligns with renal diet guidelines.

Ingredients:

- 1 block extra-firm tofu, pressed and cubed
- 2 tablespoons soy sauce (low-sodium)
- 1 tablespoon sesame oil
- 1 tablespoon olive oil
- 1 bell pepper, thinly sliced
- 1 carrot, julienned
- 1 cup broccoli florets
- 1 cup snap peas, trimmed
- 3 green onions, sliced
- 2 cloves garlic, minced
- 1 teaspoon fresh ginger, grated
- Sesame seeds, for garnish

Instructions:

1. In a bowl, toss the cubed tofu with low-sodium soy sauce and let it marinate for at least 15 minutes.
2. Heat olive oil in a wok or large skillet over medium-high heat.

3. Add the marinated tofu to the skillet and cook until golden brown on all sides. Remove the tofu from the skillet and set aside.

4. In the same skillet, add sesame oil and sauté garlic and ginger until fragrant.

5. Add sliced bell pepper, julienned carrot, broccoli florets, and snap peas to the skillet. Stir-fry the vegetables until they are crisp-tender.

6. Return the cooked tofu to the skillet and add sliced green onions. Toss everything together until well combined.

7. Garnish the vegetable stir-fry with sesame seeds and serve over brown rice or a kidney-friendly grain of your choice.

Practical Tip: Feel free to customize the vegetable stir-fry with other kidney-friendly vegetables such as zucchini, mushrooms, or bok choy. Adjust the level of spiciness by adding red pepper flakes or chili sauce according to your taste preferences. This versatile stir-fry offers a delicious way to incorporate a variety of plant-based ingredients into your renal diet.

8.3 Lentil and Vegetable Stew

Lentils are a nutritious and high-fiber legume that can be the star of a hearty and kidney-friendly vegetable stew. Packed with protein and essential nutrients, this stew is a comforting and satisfying dinner option that aligns with renal diet guidelines.

Ingredients:

- 1 cup dry green or brown lentils, rinsed and drained
- 1 tablespoon olive oil
- 1 onion, diced
- 2 carrots, diced
- 2 celery stalks, diced
- 3 cloves garlic, minced
- 1 teaspoon ground cumin
- 1 teaspoon ground coriander
- 1/2 teaspoon smoked paprika
- 1 bay leaf
- 4 cups low-sodium vegetable broth
- 1 can (14 ounces) diced tomatoes (low-sodium)
- 2 cups kale or spinach, chopped
- Salt and pepper, to taste
- Fresh parsley, for garnish

Instructions:

1. In a large pot, heat olive oil over medium heat.
2. Add diced onion, carrots, and celery to the pot. Sauté until the vegetables are softened.

3. Add minced garlic, ground cumin, ground coriander, smoked paprika, and bay leaf to the pot. Stir to coat the vegetables with the spices.

4. Pour in low-sodium vegetable broth and add rinsed lentils. Bring the mixture to a boil.

5. Reduce the heat to simmer, cover the pot, and let it cook for about 25-30 minutes or until the lentils are tender.

6. Add diced tomatoes and chopped kale or spinach to the pot. Stir well and let it simmer for an additional 5-7 minutes.

7. Season the stew with salt and pepper to taste. Remove the bay leaf.

8. Serve the lentil and vegetable stew hot, garnished with fresh parsley.

Practical Tip: This lentil and vegetable stew can be prepared in advance and stored in the refrigerator for convenient and quick dinners throughout the week. Consider adding kidney-friendly herbs, such as thyme or rosemary, for additional flavor. Serve the stew over a small portion of cooked quinoa or whole grain rice for a well-rounded and satisfying meal.

These dinner recipes follow the guidelines of a renal diet, but they also provide a range of flavors and nutritional advantages. You may have tasty and nutritious dinners that promote kidney health by combining lean proteins, kidney-friendly veggies, and well chosen seasonings. Feel free to modify these recipes as you try them to fit your dietary requirements and taste preferences, ensuring a delightful and long-lasting renal diet experience.

Chapter 9: Snacks and Sides

Satisfying snacks and delectable sides can liven up your renal diet in between meals and keep you full and active all day. Three delicious meals that mix taste, nutrition, and renal diet recommendations are covered in this chapter: Guacamole, Fresh Fruit Skewers, and Roasted Chickpeas served with Homemade Renal-Friendly Chips.

9.1 Roasted Chickpeas

Roasted chickpeas are a crunchy and protein-packed snack that makes a delightful addition to your renal diet. These little powerhouses are not only satisfying but also customizable with various seasonings, allowing you to experiment with different flavor profiles.

Ingredients:

- 1 can (15 ounces) chickpeas, drained and rinsed
- 1 tablespoon olive oil
- 1/2 teaspoon ground cumin
- 1/2 teaspoon smoked paprika

- 1/4 teaspoon garlic powder

- Salt and pepper, to taste

Instructions:

1. Preheat the oven to 400°F (200°C).

2. Pat the drained chickpeas dry with a paper towel to remove excess moisture.

3. In a bowl, toss the chickpeas with olive oil, ground cumin, smoked paprika, garlic powder, salt, and pepper until evenly coated.

4. Spread the seasoned chickpeas in a single layer on a baking sheet lined with parchment paper.

5. Roast in the preheated oven for 20-25 minutes or until the chickpeas are golden brown and crispy, shaking the pan halfway through to ensure even cooking.

6. Remove from the oven and let the roasted chickpeas cool before serving.

Practical Tip: Experiment with different spice combinations to create a variety of roasted chickpea flavors. You can try options like chili powder, curry seasoning, or a touch of lemon zest. Keep a batch on hand for a convenient and kidney-friendly snack that satisfies your crunchy cravings.

9.2 Fresh Fruit Skewers

Fresh fruit skewers provide a colorful and refreshing snack that combines the natural sweetness of various fruits. This snack is not only visually appealing but also packed with vitamins, minerals, and antioxidants, making it a delightful addition to your renal diet.

Ingredients:

- 1 cup watermelon, cubed
- 1 cup pineapple, cubed
- 1 cup strawberries, hulled
- 1 cup grapes, red or green
- Wooden skewers

Instructions:

1. Prepare the fruit by washing and cutting the watermelon, pineapple, strawberries, and grapes into bite-sized pieces.
2. Thread the fruit pieces onto wooden skewers in a colorful and appealing pattern.
3. Arrange the fruit skewers on a serving platter.

Practical Tip: Feel free to customize the fruit selection based on your preferences and seasonal availability. For added variety, you can include low-potassium options such as apple slices, melon, or kiwi. Serve the fresh fruit skewers chilled for a refreshing and hydrating snack.

9.3 Guacamole with Homemade Renal-Friendly Chips

Guacamole is a creamy and flavorful dip that can be enjoyed with homemade renal-friendly chips. Avocados provide healthy fats while the homemade chips offer a satisfying crunch. This snack is not only delicious but also easy to prepare, making it a perfect addition to your renal diet repertoire.

Ingredients:

For Guacamole:

- 2 ripe avocados, peeled and pitted
- 1 medium tomato, diced
- 1/4 cup red onion, finely chopped
- 1 clove garlic, minced
- 1 tablespoon fresh cilantro, chopped
- 1 tablespoon lime juice
- Salt and pepper, to taste

For Homemade Renal-Friendly Chips:

- 4 whole-grain or low-sodium tortillas
- Olive oil cooking spray
- Salt, to taste

Instructions:

For Guacamole:

1. In a bowl, mash the ripe avocados with a fork.
2. Add diced tomato, chopped red onion, minced garlic, chopped fresh cilantro, lime juice, salt, and pepper to the mashed avocados. Mix until well combined.
3. Adjust salt and pepper to taste, and set the guacamole aside.

For Homemade Renal-Friendly Chips:

1. Preheat the oven to 350°F (175°C).
2. Stack the tortillas and cut them into triangles.
3. Arrange the tortilla triangles in a single layer on a baking sheet.
4. Lightly coat the tortilla triangles with olive oil cooking spray and sprinkle with a pinch of salt.
5. Bake in the preheated oven for 8-10 minutes or until the chips are golden brown and crispy.

6. Remove the chips from the oven and let them cool before serving.

Practical Tip: Experiment with additional ingredients in your guacamole, such as diced jalapeños or a touch of cumin, to add depth and flavor. Ensure the tortillas are crispy but not overly browned to avoid excessive sodium content. This snack provides a balance of creamy and crunchy textures, making it a delightful treat for any time of day.

While following the guidelines of a renal diet, these snacks and sides provide a variety of flavors and textures. You can enjoy tasty and filling snacks that promote kidney health by combining healthful ingredients, low-sodium spices, and kidney-friendly alternatives. Feel free to customize any of these recipes as you try them out based on your dietary requirements and taste preferences to make your journey toward a sustainable and pleasurable renal diet.

Chapter 10: Desserts with a Kidney-Friendly Twist

Not only is it feasible to satisfy your sweet appetite while following the guidelines of a renal diet, but it's also enjoyable. This chapter will cover three delectable dessert dishes that update beloved classics in a kidney-friendly way: Angel Food Cake with Fresh Fruit, Chia Seed Pudding with Almond Milk, and Berry Sorbet.

10.1 Berry Sorbet

Refreshing and bursting with natural fruit flavors, berry sorbet offers a cool and satisfying way to indulge in a sweet treat without compromising your renal diet. This simple and delightful dessert is a perfect finale to any meal.

Ingredients:

- 2 cups mixed berries (such as strawberries, blueberries, and raspberries)
- 1/4 cup water
- 1/4 cup honey or maple syrup
- 1 tablespoon fresh lemon juice
- Mint leaves, for garnish (optional)

Instructions:

1. Rinse and prepare the mixed berries, removing stems and hulls as needed.
2. In a blender or food processor, combine the mixed berries, water, honey or maple syrup, and fresh lemon juice.
3. Blend until smooth, scraping down the sides as needed to ensure all ingredients are well incorporated.
4. Taste the mixture and adjust sweetness or acidity if needed by adding more honey or lemon juice.
5. Pour the sorbet mixture into a shallow dish or ice cube trays.
6. Freeze for about 4-6 hours, stirring or blending the mixture every hour to prevent ice crystals from forming.
7. Once the sorbet has reached a firm consistency, scoop it into serving bowls or glasses.
8. Garnish with mint leaves if desired and serve immediately.

Practical Tip: Experiment with different berry combinations to discover your favorite flavor profile. For added texture, you can fold in whole berries before freezing. This berry sorbet provides a refreshing and guilt-free way to indulge in a sweet dessert that aligns with your renal diet.

10.2 Angel Food Cake with Fresh Fruit

Light, airy, and paired with fresh fruit, this kidney-friendly version of Angel Food Cake brings a touch of elegance to your dessert repertoire. Enjoy the delightful combination of fluffy cake and vibrant fruit for a satisfying and guilt-free treat.

Ingredients:

For Angel Food Cake:

- 1 cup cake flour
- 1 1/2 cups egg whites (approximately 10-12 large eggs)
- 1 1/2 teaspoons cream of tartar
- 1 cup granulated sugar
- 1 teaspoon vanilla extract
- 1/4 teaspoon almond extract
- 1/4 teaspoon salt

For Fresh Fruit Topping:

- 2 cups mixed fresh berries (such as strawberries, blueberries, and raspberries)
- 1 tablespoon honey or maple syrup
- Fresh mint leaves, for garnish (optional)

Instructions:

For Angel Food Cake:

1. Preheat the oven to 350°F (175°C).
2. Sift cake flour and set aside.
3. In a large, clean, and dry mixing bowl, whip egg whites and cream of tartar until soft peaks form.
4. Gradually add granulated sugar, one tablespoon at a time, while continuing to whip the egg whites until glossy and stiff peaks form.
5. Gently fold in vanilla extract, almond extract, and salt.
6. Sift the cake flour over the egg white mixture in small batches, folding gently to incorporate without deflating the egg whites.
7. Spoon the batter into an ungreased Angel Food Cake pan and smooth the top.
8. Bake in the preheated oven for 35-40 minutes or until the top is golden brown and the cake springs back when touched.
9. Invert the cake pan onto a cooling rack and let it cool completely.

For Fresh Fruit Topping:

1. Rinse and prepare the mixed berries, removing stems and hulls as needed.

2. In a bowl, gently toss the mixed berries with honey or maple syrup until well coated.

3. Allow the berries to macerate for a few minutes to release their natural juices.

4. Slice the cooled Angel Food Cake and serve with a generous spoonful of fresh berries on top.

5. Garnish with fresh mint leaves if desired and serve.

Practical Tip: Angel Food Cake is naturally low in fat, and using a sugar substitute can help manage sugar intake. Consider serving this dessert with a dollop of kidney-friendly whipped cream made from non-dairy alternatives. This light and fruity dessert provide a delightful way to conclude your meal with a kidney-friendly sweet treat.

10.3 Chia Seed Pudding with Almond Milk

Chia seed pudding is a versatile and nutrient-packed dessert that aligns perfectly with a renal diet. By using almond milk and incorporating your favorite toppings, you can create a satisfying and customizable treat that is rich in fiber, omega-3 fatty acids, and essential nutrients.

Ingredients:

- 1/4 cup chia seeds
- 1 cup unsweetened almond milk (low-potassium)
- 1 tablespoon honey or maple syrup
- 1/2 teaspoon vanilla extract
- Fresh fruit, nuts, or seeds for topping

Instructions:

1. In a bowl, combine chia seeds, unsweetened almond milk, honey or maple syrup, and vanilla extract.
2. Whisk the ingredients together until well combined.
3. Cover the bowl and refrigerate for at least 4 hours or overnight to allow the chia seeds to absorb the liquid and create a pudding-like consistency.
4. Stir the chia seed pudding before serving to ensure an even texture.
5. Spoon the pudding into individual serving glasses or bowls.
6. Top with your choice of fresh fruit, nuts, or seeds for added flavor and texture.

Practical Tip: Experiment with different toppings to create diverse flavor profiles for your chia seed pudding. Consider using low-potassium fruits such as berries, kiwi, or pineapple. This versatile dessert provides a satisfying and nutritious option that is easy to prepare and can be customized to suit your taste preferences.

While following the guidelines of a renal diet, these sweets are suitable for people with kidneys and offer a variety of flavors and textures. You can enjoy tasty and fulfilling sweet sweets that support kidney health by using fresh, low-potassium products and practicing careful portion control. Feel free to modify these recipes as you try them to fit your dietary requirements and taste preferences, ensuring a delightful and long-lasting renal diet experience.

Chapter 11: Dining Out and Special Occasions

Giving up eating out or special occasion celebrations is not necessary while starting a renal diet. It is possible to manage kidney disease and still enjoy tasty meals with a little planning and attention to detail. This chapter will discuss helpful ways to navigate restaurant menus and offer advice on how to celebrate without endangering renal health.

11.1 Navigating Restaurant Menus

When dining out, a renal diet calls for a planned and knowledgeable approach. Even though restaurant menus can be intimidating, there are a few important factors to keep in mind while making decisions that support your renal health objectives.

1. Familiarize Yourself with Menu Terminology

It's essential to comprehend menu language in order to make wise decisions. The following terms should be understood:

- **Broiling:** An approach to cooking that applies direct heat from above. For a healthier choice, go with broiled instead than fried food.

- **Grilled:** Using direct heat, frequently over an open flame, grilling is similar to broiling. In general, grilled foods are a good option, but watch out for overly salty or marinated foods.

- **Steamed:** Steam-cooked food maintains its original flavors and nutrients. Select protein or steamed veggies for a kidney-friendly meal.

- **Baked:** Baking is a healthier substitute for frying since it uses dry heat. On the menu, look for baked alternatives.

- **Poached:** Poaching is the process of preparing food by slowly simmering it in liquid. Poached foods frequently have reduced fat and salt content.

- **Reduced Sodium:** Certain dishes may be served in lower-sodium variants at some establishments. Never be afraid to inquire about adapted recipes.

2. Choose Lean Proteins

A renal diet must include protein, but the type of protein you eat must be lean. Think about the following options for proteins when dining out:

- **Chicken Breast:** Lean and kidney-friendly options include skinless, grilled, or baked chicken breast.

- **Fish:** Fish that has been baked or grilled, like tilapia or salmon, delivers omega-3 fatty acids without having too much sodium.

- **Lean Cuts of Meat:** Select lean beef or pig cuts and use broiling or grilling as your technique of preparation.

- **Plant-Based Proteins:** Look into plant-based protein sources including quinoa, tofu, and lentils.

3. Be Mindful of Sodium

One of the most important aspects of controlling renal illness is diet. Remember the following when dining out:

- **Requesting Modifications:** Do not be afraid to ask for adjustments to your meal, including requesting for dressings or sauces to be served separately. You now have more control over how much sodium you eat.

- **Choosing Fresh Ingredients:** Since fresh produce is naturally low in sodium, choose dishes that feature it.

- **Avoiding Processed Foods:** Because they frequently contain a lot of sodium, avoid eating processed or cured meats.

4. Control Portion Sizes

Portion sizes at many restaurants are larger than suggested by diets. To control serving sizes:

- **Sharing Dishes:** To cut down on the quantity of food on your plate, think about splitting a dinner with a dining partner.

- **Choosing Appetizers:** As your main course, go for starters or appetizers. They frequently arrive in smaller servings.

- **Taking Home Leftovers:** Don't be afraid to request a container to take leftovers home if the servings are big.

5. Hydration is Key

Kidney health depends on maintaining adequate fluids. When eating at a restaurant:

- **Limiting Coffee and Alcohol:** Dehydration can be exacerbated by both caffeine and alcohol. Choose herbal tea, water, or other non-alcoholic, non-caffeinated liquids.

- **Bring a Water Bottle:** To make sure you have access to water during your lunch, think about bringing a reusable water bottle.

- **Choosing Low-Potassium Beverages:** If you're worried about your potassium intake, go for drinks that have less potassium in them.

6. Dessert Considerations

Dessert is OK if you make some thoughtful decisions:

- Fruit-Based Desserts: Sorbet or fresh fruit can make filling, kidney-friendly desserts.
- Portion Control: Request a smaller portion or split desserts with others.
- Avoiding High-Potassium Options: Desserts with high-potassium components should be avoided if potassium is an issue.

11.2 Tips for Celebrating without Compromising Kidney Health

Festivities and special occasions are moments to enjoy delectable cuisine and companionship. It's crucial to enjoy life sensibly when treating kidney disease. The following advice will help you enjoy special events without jeopardizing your kidneys' health:

1. Plan Ahead

Think about the following before going to a celebration or special event:

- **Communication:** Let the host or restaurant know ahead of time about any dietary requirements or preferences.
- **Research the Menu:** Try to choose selections that are kidney-friendly by looking over the menu in advance.
- **Eat a Snack**: Before the event, consuming a small, kidney-friendly snack will help suppress your hunger and lessen the temptation to indulge in less healthful choices.

2. Bring a Dish

Think about bringing a meal that is kidney-friendly to contribute if you're going to a potluck or get-together. This guarantees that you always have a healthy choice on hand and shares delectable renal diet dishes with others.

3. Mindful Eating

You can appreciate special times more when you eat mindfully:

- **Savor Each Bite:** Give your food enough time to develop taste. You can learn to detect when you're full by eating gently.
- **Stay Hydrated:** To stay hydrated during the event, sip water.
- **Be Selective:** Rather of trying everything on the menu, pick a few exceptional dishes that you really like.

4. Be Assertive but Polite

It's critical to express your demands to others while maintaining a renal diet without feeling self-conscious:

- **Politely Decline:** When offered food that doesn't fit your diet, gently say "no" and explain why you are following certain dietary restrictions.
- **Ask Questions:** Never be afraid to question servers or hosts about ingredients or cooking techniques.

5. Watch Sodium Intake

Meals on special occasions may consist more of restaurant- or processed food items, which may have more sodium:

- **Requesting Modifications:** Ask for lower-sodium alternatives and sauces and dressings on the side.
- **Limiting Processed Foods:** Choose whole, fresh foods over processed or pre-packaged options.

6. Continue Your Exercise

Even on special occasions, engaging in physical activity is essential to living a healthy lifestyle:

- **Plan Activities:** To counterbalance the celebration dinner, recommend physically demanding activities like a stroll or outdoor games.
- **Encourage Others:** Invite loved ones to participate with you in physical activities.

7. Choose Wisely

Celebrate while maintaining renal health by making well-considered decisions:

- **Balanced Plate**: A balanced plate should include a variety of fresh vegetables, complete grains, and lean proteins.
- **Portion Control**: Pay attention to how much you eat, particularly when there are lots of delicious options available.
- **Enjoy the Moment**: Don't just concentrate on the food; instead, enjoy the company and the happiness of the occasion.

8. Dessert Alternatives

For a delicious, kidney-friendly way to cap off a wonderful dinner:

- **Fresh Fruit:** For a cool dessert, go for a fruit salad or a dish of fresh fruit.

- **Customized Desserts:** Try to bring or ask for a dessert option that is kidney-friendly.
- **Moderation is Key:** Eat dessert in moderation, taking pleasure in every bite.

It is still possible to have pleasant celebrations of key occasions while putting renal health first. Planning ahead, making thoughtful decisions, and keeping lines of communication open will help you enjoy excellent meals and navigate social gatherings without sacrificing your renal diet objectives. Recall that every occasion presents a chance to highlight tasty and nutritious kidney-friendly substitutes.

Chapter 12: Staying Hydrated: The Importance of Fluid Management

An essential component of renal health, proper hydration supports both general health and kidney function. This chapter will examine the importance of fluid management for people with kidney illness, including strategies for tracking fluid consumption and helpful hydration advice catered to the special requirements of renal patients.

12.1 Monitoring Fluid Intake

Monitoring fluid intake is crucial for renal disease patients in order to maintain a balance that promotes good kidney function. The kidneys are essential for controlling the body's fluid balance; therefore monitoring fluid intake closely becomes critical when renal function is impaired.

1. Understanding Fluid Balance

The equilibrium between the body's fluid intake and output is referred to as fluid balance. For renal patients, achieving and maintaining appropriate fluid balance is essential to avoiding problems from dehydration or fluid retention.

- **Fluid Intake:** This refers to the consumption of any liquid, including drinks and foods high in moisture, such as soups and fruits.
- **Fluid Output:** The body expels fluids by breathing, sweating, and peeing.

2. Recommended Fluid Intake

The amount of fluid that is advised can change depending on a number of variables, including age, gender, climate, and personal health issues. Although there isn't a single, universally applicable guideline for kidney patients, medical professionals frequently customize suggestions depending on the unique requirements of each patient.

- **General Guideline**: It is generally advised to drink about 8 cups (64 ounces) of fluid each day in order to maintain fluid balance. This can, however, differ.
- **Individualized Approach:** Recipients may get tailored advice according to their kidney disease stage, general health, and individual symptoms.

3. Importance of Monitoring

For renal patients, keeping an eye on their fluid intake is essential to avoiding problems brought on by fluid imbalance. Principal rationales for tracking fluid consumption consist of:

- **Fluid Restriction:** In order to prevent fluid overload and its associated problems, some people with advanced renal disease may need to restrict their fluid intake.
- **Dehydration Prevention:** Conversely, insufficient consumption of fluids can result in dehydration, which may give rise to complications such electrolyte abnormalities.
- **Symptom Management:** Monitoring fluid intake can aid in the management of symptoms such as high blood pressure and edema, or the retention of fluid.

4. Signs of Fluid Imbalance

Kidney sufferers must be alert for any indications of fluid imbalance. Typical indicators consist of:

- **Edema:** Fluid retention may be indicated by swelling in the legs, ankles, or other regions of the body.
- **Shortness of Breath:** An accumulation of fluid in the lungs can cause dyspnea.

- **Changes in Urination:** It's important to keep an eye on any variations in the amount, color, or frequency of urine produced. Dehydration may be indicated by decreased urine production or dark urine.
- **High Blood Pressure:** Retention of fluids may be a factor in high blood pressure.

12.2 Hydration Tips for Kidney Patients

For those with renal illness, staying properly hydrated requires a careful balance. Kidney patients can enjoy an appropriate fluid intake while avoiding the difficulties linked to fluid excess by putting these helpful hydration suggestions into practice. The following particular advice is designed with renal patients' particular needs in mind:

1. Consult Your Healthcare Team

Personalized advice from your medical team is crucial for controlling how much fluid you consume. To make recommendations that are unique to you, your healthcare professional can evaluate your kidney function, overall health, and any current conditions.

- **Regular Check-Ups**: Make routine visits with your nephrologist or other healthcare practitioner to check kidney function and obtain the most recent recommendations regarding fluid management.

2. Be Mindful of Sodium Intake

Since sodium is essential for maintaining fluid balance, it is critical for kidney patients to watch how much sodium they consume. While moderate sodium consumption promotes appropriate fluid balance, excessive sodium can lead to fluid retention.

- **Read Labels:** Read the labels and take note of the salt level in processed and packaged goods. Choose options that are salt-free or low in sodium.
- **Use Herbs and Spices:** Instead of using salt as a seasoning, add flavor to your food by using herbs and spices.
- **Limit Processed Foods:** Because processed and quick foods frequently include excessive salt levels, reduce your intake of them.

3. Choose Hydrating Foods

Adding items that are high in water content to your diet will help you consume more fluids and get extra nutrients. Among the foods that are hydrating are:

- **Cucumber:** Cucumber, which has high water content, is a pleasant snack on its own or a great addition to salads.
- **Watermelon:** Not only is it a tasty summertime treat, but water makes up the majority of its content.
- **Berries:** In addition to being high in antioxidants, raspberries, blueberries, and strawberries also help to keep you hydrated overall.
- **Soups and Broths:** A hydrating option would be to include soups made with vegetables that are high in moisture content and low in sodium.

4. Monitor Fluid Intake and Output

Monitoring your fluid intake and output will assist you in keeping a healthy balance. Take into account these suggestions:

- **Use a Journal:** Keep track of the kinds and quantities of fluids you consume throughout the day by keeping a fluid intake journal.
- **Monitor Urine Output:** Keep an eye out for variations in the amount, color, and frequency of pee. Should you observe any notable differences, speak with your healthcare professional.

- **Weigh Yourself:** Keep a regular eye on your weight since sharp variations could point to dehydration or fluid retention.

5. Space out Fluid Intake

Consider distributing your fluid consumption throughout the day as an alternative to ingesting big amounts at once. This method promotes a more stable fluid balance and lessens the likelihood of unexpected fluid overload.

- **Small, Frequent Sips:** Drink liquids frequently and gradually as opposed to ingesting a lot at once.
- **Set Reminders:** Remind yourself to drink water on a regular basis by setting alarms or reminders.

6. Choose Kidney-Friendly Beverages

It's critical to choose drinks that complement your renal diet if you want to keep your kidneys healthy. Choose kidney-friendly alternatives, like:

- **Water:** The purest form of hydration, pure water promotes general health and is additive-free.
- **Herbal Tea:** For a tasty and hydrating substitute, go for herbal teas that are caffeine-free.

- **Freshly Squeezed Juices**: A homemade juice produced with low-potassium fruits, such as berries or apples, might be a good way to stay hydrated.
- **Diluted Sports Drinks**: To restore electrolytes without going overboard with sodium, think about diluting sports drinks if your doctor recommends it.

7. Be Mindful of Weather and Activity Levels

Fluid requirements are influenced by physical activity and environmental conditions. Adapt your fluid intake according to your exercise level and other factors like temperature.

- **Hot Weather:** Drink more fluids in the heat to make up for the extra fluids lost through perspiration.
- **Physical Activity:** Drink plenty of water while exercising, but be aware of your own personal fluid requirements to prevent dehydration.

8. Hydration During Dialysis

Controlling fluid intake becomes even more important for dialysis patients. Dialysis aids in the body's removal of excess fluid, however it is crucial to follow fluid limitations in between sessions.

- **Follow Dialysis Guidelines:** On days when you are not receiving dialysis, abide by the fluid recommendations made by your medical team.

- **Limit High-Potassium Beverages:** To prevent consuming too much potassium, opt for low-potassium drinks.

- **Space Fluid Intake:** To avoid abrupt fluid fluctuations, space out your fluid intake equally between dialysis sessions.

9. Be Cautious with Alcohol and Caffeine

Caffeine and alcohol can both affect renal function and fluid balance. Some people may be able to consume in moderation, but others may need to use caution.

- **Moderate Consumption:** If your doctor has given the all-clear, keep your intake of alcohol and caffeine to a minimum.

- **Stay Hydrated:** Take plenty of water in addition to alcohol or caffeinated drinks in moderation.

10. Seek Support

Maintaining fluid intake while treating kidney illness might be difficult, but getting help can really help.

- **Connect with Others:** Participating in forums or support groups where people exchange stories and advice on how to control fluid consumption might yield insightful information.

- **Involve Family and Friends:** Tell everyone in your immediate vicinity about your fluid limitations and ask for their cooperation and understanding.

11. Address Thirst Wisely

While being thirsty is a normal sign that your body needs fluids, renal patients must take caution when quenching their thirst.

- **Monitor Thirst Levels:** Be mindful of your body's cues, but don't use thirst as your only indicator of dehydration.

- **Sip, Don't Chug:** To prevent a rapid intake of fluid, sip steadily rather than consuming big amounts at once.

- **Select Kidney-Friendly Options:** Make sure your hydration choices are in line with your renal diet.

In summary

Adopting workable fluid management measures is essential for renal patients, as staying hydrated is a basic part of controlling kidney illness. People with renal illness can maintain optimal kidney function and general well-being by keeping an eye on their fluid intake, selecting foods high in water content, and according to specific instructions from healthcare professionals. By putting these hydration suggestions into practice, renal patients can find a balance between getting enough fluids and avoiding problems brought on by fluid imbalance. Remember that receiving individualized advice from your healthcare team is essential to achieving optimal fluid management as you set out on your quest to maintain your kidney health and keep hydrated.

Chapter 13: Exercise and Lifestyle Considerations

The key to controlling renal disease is continuing a healthy lifestyle. This chapter will address the importance of including physical activity in your routine in a safe manner as well as stress-reduction techniques that are specifically designed to support kidney health.

13.1 Incorporating Physical Activity Safely

A healthy lifestyle must include physical activity since it improves general health and supports kidney function. To ensure that exercise is both safe and effective, there are a few things to bear in mind for those who are managing kidney illness.

1. Exercise's Advantages for Kidney Health

Regular physical activity provides many advantages for those with renal disease:

- **Cardiovascular Health:** Physical activity enhances cardiovascular health by lowering the chance of heart-related problems, which are frequently linked to kidney illness.

- **Weight management:** Exercise has a role in helping people maintain a healthy weight, which is essential for kidney health.

- **Blood Pressure Control:** Exercise on a regular basis aids in blood pressure regulation, which is crucial for kidney function.

- **Blood Sugar Regulation:** Exercise helps control blood sugar in those with diabetes, a major comorbidity of kidney disease.

- **Better Mood:** Engaging in physical activity releases endorphins, which uplift the spirit and aid in stress and anxiety reduction.

2. Consultation with Healthcare Providers

It is crucial to speak with your primary care physician or nephrologist as well as the rest of your healthcare team before starting any exercise program. Based on your unique health situation, renal function, and any current difficulties, they can offer tailored advice.

- **Individualized Recommendations:** Medical professionals can design an exercise regimen specifically for you based on your kidney disease stage, general health, and any limitations.
- **Monitoring Kidney Function:** Regular check-ups with your medical team enable continuous kidney function monitoring and necessary modifications to activity suggestions.

3. Types of Exercise for Kidney Patients

For renal patients, selecting the appropriate forms of exercise is essential to ensuring safety and efficacy. Think about include any of the following workouts in your regimen:

- **Aerobic Exercise:** Exercises that don't overly tax the kidneys, such as walking, cycling, swimming, or low-impact aerobics, are good for the heart.
- **Strength Training:** Including mild to moderate strength training activities can enhance general function and muscle strength. But it's important to stay away from big weights and undue pressure.

- **Stretching and Flexibility:** Mild stretches improve range of motion, lower the chance of injury, and increase flexibility.
- **Mind-Body Exercises**: Activities that combine physical activity with stress-reduction strategies, like yoga or tai chi, are beneficial for both mental and physical health.

4. Exercise Frequency and Duration

Kidney patients should exercise moderately and consistently when it comes to how often and how long they exercise:

- **Consistent Routine:** Try to stick to a regular fitness schedule that incorporates a variety of strength, flexibility, and cardio workouts.
- **Gradual Progression:** As your fitness level increases, start with shorter workouts and lower intensity and progressively increase.
- **Listen to Your Body:** Be mindful of how your body reacts to exercise and refrain from overexerting yourself.

5. Hydration During Exercise

It's important to be properly hydrated during exercising, especially if you have renal disease:

- **Fluid consumption Considerations:** Discuss specific guidelines for fluid consumption during exercise with your healthcare professional.
- **Avoid Over hydration:** Although it's important to stay hydrated, too much water can put stress on the kidneys. Adjust your hydration intake based on your sweat rate and personal demands.

6. Temperature Considerations

It's important for kidney patients, especially those on dialysis, to take their temperature into account when exercising:

- **Avoid Extreme Temperatures:** While excessive cold can present additional obstacles, high temperatures can cause dehydration. If the weather is bad, choose to workout indoors.
- **Dialysis Timing:** To prevent putting further stress on your body, if you receive dialysis, think about planning your activity on days when you don't receive it.

7. Monitoring Symptoms

The secret to maintaining safety when exercising understands how your body reacts to it:

- **Watch for Warning Signs:** Keep an eye out for signs including unusual exhaustion, chest pain, dizziness, and shortness of breath. You should cease exercising and speak with your doctor if any of these happen.
- **Adapt as Needed:** Adapt your fitness regimen to your current state of health on a particular day. It's acceptable to change the time or intensity to suit your energy levels.

8. Group Exercise and Social Support

Getting social support or participating in group exercise might improve your overall experience of adding physical activity to your routine:

- **Joining Classes:** Group exercise classes or programs tailored to the needs of people with chronic illnesses can offer a supportive setting.
- **Buddy System:** Working out with a buddy or relative adds an extra degree of support in addition to making the exercise more fun.
- **Community Resources:** Look into the available local resources that provide specialized fitness regimens for people with renal illness.

9. Adaptations for Specific Stages of Kidney Disease

The following exercise guidelines may change depending on the stage of renal disease:

- **Early Stages:** People with kidney disease may experience less limitation and have greater flexibility in their workout regimen.
- **Advanced Stages:** Exercise suggestions may be more individualized and adjustments may be required for individuals in advanced stages or receiving dialysis.
- **Individualized Guidance:** Collaborate closely with your medical team to obtain tailored advice and modifications according to your unique circumstances.

13.2 Stress Management for Kidney Health

In addition to being essential for preserving general wellbeing, stress management is also critical for preserving renal health in those with kidney disease. Prolonged stress can aggravate associated disorders and accelerate the course of renal disease. As a result, implementing efficient stress-reduction techniques is crucial for a thorough approach to kidney care.

1. The Impact of Stress on Kidney Health

Stress sets off a physiological reaction in the body that can impact the kidneys among other systems:

- **Elevated Blood Pressure**: Prolonged stress can lead to high blood pressure, which further strains the kidneys.

- **Inflammation:** Stress may be a factor in inflammation, which can have a detrimental effect on kidney function.

- **Behavioral Factors:** Stress can affect actions that have an adverse effect on kidney health, such eating poorly, getting too little sleep, and engaging in less physical exercise.

2. Stress-Reducing Techniques

Including stress-reduction methods in your everyday practice will help improve your general health and kidney health:

- **Mindfulness Meditation**: Techniques for mindful meditation, such guided meditation or focused breathing, can help people unwind and cope with stress.

- **Yoga and Tai Chi:** These mind-body practices offer a comprehensive approach to stress treatment by fusing physical activity with relaxation techniques.

- **Progressive Muscle Relaxation:** This method encourages both physical and mental calm by gradually tensing and relaxing various muscle groups.

- **Deep Breathing Exercises:** By triggering the body's relaxation response, slow, deep breathing can help reduce stress.

- **Nature Walks:** It has been demonstrated that spending time in nature, whether on a hike or a stroll in a park, lowers stress levels.

3. Lifestyle Modifications for Stress Reduction

Certain lifestyle changes, in addition to certain stress-reduction methods, can help with overall stress management:

- **Adequate Sleep:** Make high quality sleep a priority because it's essential for both stress relief and general health.
- **Balanced Nutrition:** Eating a diet that is friendly to the kidneys promotes general health as well as kidney health.
- **Regular Exercise:** Exercise has been shown to have a number of positive health impacts, including reducing stress.
- **Social Connections:** Keeping up good social ties with friends and family offers stress management and emotional support.

4. Seeking Professional Support

For certain people, seeking professional assistance in stress management may be necessary.

- **Counseling or therapy:** Consulting with a mental health expert might yield insightful information and stress-reduction techniques.

- **Support Groups:** Participating in support groups for people with kidney disease or other chronic illnesses helps foster a feeling of shared experience and community.

- **Mind-Body Programs:** Attending organized mind-body events, such stress management seminars, might provide you useful coping mechanisms.

5. Balancing Responsibilities

Managing stress requires striking a balance between different life commitments.

- **Time management:** To lessen emotions of overwhelm, prioritize your work, assign assignments when you can, and use time management techniques.

- **Setting Realistic Goals:** Take into account your general health and well-being when setting realistic objectives for yourself.

- **Learning to Say No:** Be aware of your boundaries and don't be afraid to turn down requests for more work when necessary.

6. Creating a Relaxation Routine

Including relaxation exercises in your weekly or daily routine can help you manage stress over time:

- **Scheduled Breaks:** Throughout the day, set aside brief periods of time to practice relaxation techniques such as deep breathing, stretching, or brief meditation.
- **Regular Leisure Activities:** Set aside time for enjoyable pursuits, such as reading, listening to music, or taking up a hobby.
- **Nature Connection:** Even a brief period of time spent outside can be soothing when spent in the great outdoors.

7. Mindful Eating for Stress Reduction

Eating mindfully entails being in the present moment and focusing on the sensory aspects of the meal, this exercise can enhance general wellbeing and help reduce stress:

- **Slow and Enjoyable Meals:** Give your meal enough time to develop flavors and textures as you relish each bite.
- **Avoid Multitasking:** To improve the mindful eating experience, reduce outside distractions during meals, such as watching television or working.

- **Gratitude Practice:** Develop a positive relationship with food by being grateful for the sustenance your meals bring.

8. Balancing Work and Rest

For effective stress management, finding the ideal balance between work and relaxation is essential.

- **Regular Breaks:** Schedule little periods of time during the workday to stretch, move, or practice relaxation techniques.
- **Setting Boundaries:** To avoid burnout, clearly define the limits between work and personal time.
- **Prioritizing Self-Care:** Give self-care a high priority and acknowledge the value of relaxation and renewal.

In summary

A comprehensive strategy to controlling renal illness must include safe physical exercise and the use of appropriate stress management techniques. You can improve your overall well-being and promote kidney health by working with your healthcare team, practicing stress-reduction measures, and engaging in appropriate activity. Recall that tailored advice is essential, and your medical professionals can make tailored suggestions depending on your particular needs and state of health. In order to support your kidney health journey, prioritise consistency, gradual growth, and a holistic approach as you begin your quest to incorporate physical exercise and stress management into your lifestyle.

Chapter 14: Monitoring and Adjusting Your Renal Diet

Preparing meals is only one aspect of proactively managing your renal diet; continuous monitoring and modifications are necessary to maintain optimal kidney health. This chapter will discuss the value of routine examinations and blood work, as well as offer advice on how to modify your renal diet as needed.

14.1 Regular Check-ups and Blood Tests

Frequent evaluations by your medical team and sporadic blood tests are essential for managing renal disease properly. Regular evaluations allow medical professionals to keep an eye on your kidney function, spot any changes, and modify your treatment strategy as needed. This is why routine examinations and blood testing are so important:

1. Monitoring Kidney Function

A regular check-up with your nephrologist or other healthcare professional enables ongoing kidney function monitoring. This entails evaluating important metrics like:

- **Glomerular Filtration Rate (GFR):** This indicator shows how well your kidneys remove waste from your blood. Observing changes in GFR over time offers important information about kidney function.
- **Creatinine Levels:** The kidneys remove waste products like creatinine from the blood. Reduced renal function may be indicated by elevated creatinine levels.
- **Blood Urea Nitrogen (BUN):** This test determines how much blood contains urea nitrogen. Increased BUN levels may indicate deteriorated renal health.

2. Monitoring of Blood Pressure

One typical complication of renal illness is high blood pressure. Monitoring your blood pressure as part of routine check-ups helps you spot any swings and decide whether to change your lifestyle or medication.

- **Target Blood Pressure:** For patients with kidney disease, healthcare professionals frequently set goal blood pressure levels. The kidneys are protected when blood pressure stays within certain ranges.

- **Medication Adjustments:** To control hypertension, healthcare professionals may prescribe or modify medication based on blood pressure readings.

3. Electrolyte Balance

The body's electrolyte balance is largely maintained by the kidneys. Frequent blood tests measure electrolyte concentrations, encompassing:

- **Potassium:** Excessive potassium levels need to be closely watched since they can affect heart health.
- **Phosphorus**: Increased phosphorus levels may be linked to cardiovascular and bone problems; you may need to modify your diet or take medication.
- **Calcium:** The levels of calcium can be impacted by kidney disease, which may have an effect on bone health. Keeping an eye on calcium levels enables medical professionals to make wise recommendations.

4. Anemia Management

Anemia is a frequent side effect of kidney disease that is frequently brought on by a reduction in the kidneys' ability to generate the hormone erythropoietin. Frequent blood tests evaluate:

- **Hemoglobin Levels:** Your blood's ability to carry oxygen is indicated by your hemoglobin levels. Sustaining adequate hemoglobin levels is essential for general health.
- **Iron Levels:** The synthesis of red blood cells depends on iron. Healthcare professionals can address anemia and provide relevant interventions with the use of iron level monitoring.

5. Medication Assessment

Medication is frequently used by people with kidney disease to control blood pressure, electrolyte imbalances, and other related symptoms. Regular examinations offer the chance to:

- **Review Medications:** Medical professionals evaluate the efficacy of prescribed drugs and alter them as necessary.
- **Address Side Effects:** During check-ups, any medication-related side effects or complications can be found and dealt with.

6. Diabetes Management

For people with diabetes and kidney disease, routine examinations are crucial for controlling blood sugar levels and averting problems. Observing:

- **Blood Glucose Levels:** Monitoring blood glucose levels on a regular basis aids in maintaining ideal control and guards against additional kidney damage.
- **Hemoglobin A1c:** This test helps with long-term diabetes control by giving a snapshot of blood sugar levels over the last few months.

7. Dietary Guidance

You can talk to your healthcare team about your eating habits, difficulties, and accomplishments during routine check-ups. This conversation enables medical professionals to modify your renal diet plan and offer continuing advice.

- **Nutrient Intake Assessment:** By evaluating your nutrient intake, medical professionals can make sure you're getting the nutrients you need to stay within your limitations.
- **Addressing Challenges:** Talking about issues you have with your renal diet at check-ups enables medical professionals to provide helpful advice and modifications.

8. Emotional Well-being

Maintaining physical and mental well-being is essential for managing a chronic illness such as renal disease. Regular examinations offer the chance to:

- **Discuss Emotional Challenges:** When you are honest with your healthcare providers about any emotional difficulties or stressors you are experiencing, they can provide assistance or, if necessary, refer you to mental health specialists.

- **Quality of Life Assessment:** Assessing your total quality of life enables medical professionals to make recommendations that are in line with your preferences and way of living.

9. Treatment Plan Adjustments

Your overall treatment plan may be modified by healthcare professionals based on the data collected during routine check-ups. This may consist of:

- **Medication Changes:** Changing the kind or amount of drugs to better control anemia, blood pressure, or other associated problems.

- **Dietary Modifications:** Adapting your renal diet plan to your changing demands and circumstances while still making sure you get enough nourishment.

- **Referral to Specialists:** Should certain problems emerge, your physician may recommend that you speak with dietitians, nephrology nurses, or mental health providers.

14.2 Making Adjustments as Needed

It's a dynamic and continuous process to modify your renal diet in response to changes in kidney function, general health, or lifestyle. Being aware of when and how to make these changes gives you the ability to take an active role in the management of your kidney health. When making dietary changes, keep the following points in mind:

1. Dietary Modifications for Changing Kidney Function

Your nutritional requirements may alter as your kidney function changes over time. If you decide to modify your renal diet, take into account the following:

- **Consult with Healthcare Providers:** Get advice from your healthcare team before making any big dietary adjustments. They can offer advice depending on your overall health, kidney function right now, and dietary needs.

- **Monitor Laboratory Results:** Frequent blood tests reveal changes in renal function, electrolyte balance, and other important parameters. These findings can help you make dietary changes.

- **Fluid Restriction:** Fluid restriction may be required in kidney disease that has progressed. As recommended by your physician, modify the amount of fluids you consume.

- **Potassium Control:** Take into account modifying your consumption of foods high in potassium if your potassium levels are erratic. This can entail cutting back on or staying away from specific fruits, vegetables, and other foods high in potassium.

- **Phosphorus Management:** Dietary changes may be necessary in response to variations in phosphorus levels. Reducing the amount of foods high in phosphorus and opting for lower-phosphorus options can be advantageous.

2. Adapting to Medication Changes

Your nutritional needs may change as a result of drug additions, dose adjustments, or changes in existing prescriptions. Remain alert and make the required corrections:

Examine the Medication Instructions: Recognize how any new medications or dose adjustments may affect your diet. Certain drugs may need dietary adjustments or interact negatively with particular foods.

- **Address Side Effects:** Adjust your meal selections to account for any changes in appetite or taste perception that may result from prescription side effects.

- **Nutrient Considerations:** Be mindful of any particular dietary requirements, such as higher calcium or vitamin D intake that are related to your medications.

3. Lifestyle Changes and Dietary Adjustments

Your nutritional needs may alter as a result of lifestyle modifications like increased physical activity, weight loss, or adjustments to your daily schedule. Think about the following:

- **Increased Physical Activity:** See your healthcare provider to discuss any dietary adjustments, especially in regards to fluid and nutrient consumption, before starting a new workout regimen.

- **Weight management:** Changing the way you consume calories and distribute nutrients can help you reach and stay at a healthy weight.

- **Routine Changes:** To guarantee adherence to your renal diet, any changes to your daily schedule, such as travel or a change in meal timing, may need to be planned for and adjusted accordingly.

4. Seasonal and Environmental Factors

Your food choices can be influenced by environmental variables, such as seasonal variations and exposure to pollutants or allergens:

- **Seasonal Foods:** Modify your menus according to what fruits and veggies are in season. Eating a wide range of fresh, regional produce improves flavor and nutrition.
- **Allergies and Sensitivities:** Take into consideration any dietary decisions that may be impacted by allergies or sensitivities. To comply with these constraints, take into account modifications or replacements.

5. Psychological and Emotional Factors

Your eating habits might be influenced by your psychological well-being, stress levels, and emotional condition. Think about the following:

- **Emotional Eating:** Recognize your emotional eating habits and look for other coping strategies when facing stress or difficult emotions.
- **Celebratory Occasions:** Make plans in advance to make sure your renal diet stays on course during special events

or festivities. Look into tasty and inventive meals that are suitable for people with renal disease for these occasions.

- **Mindful Eating Practices:** Develop mindful eating practices to improve your relationship with food and your diet in general.

6. Seeking Professional Guidance

Consult experts when in doubt or faced with complicated dietary considerations:

- **Consult with a Renal Dietitian:** These professionals specialize in creating dietary plans specifically for people suffering from kidney illness. They can offer tailored advice depending on your particular requirements and preferences.

- **Engage with Mental Health Professionals:** If psychological issues have a substantial influence on your eating habits, you may want to seek out further assistance and coping mechanisms by speaking with mental health practitioners.

- **Collaborate with Healthcare Team:** Keep lines of communication open with your nephrologist, dietician, and other medical professionals. Communicate any issues or worries to get prompt, helpful support.

In summary

The dynamic process of monitoring and modifying your renal diet calls for proactive self-management as well as cooperation with your healthcare team. Effective kidney health management starts with routine examinations, blood testing, and honest dialogue with your medical professionals. You may maximize your general well-being by following dietary guidelines, being aware of changes in kidney function, and making required adjustments depending on your specific needs. Keep in mind that your medical team is an invaluable asset, providing direction and encouragement to assist you in navigating the always changing field of renal health management. As you proceed on your renal diet journey, seize the chance for development, education, and empowered decision-making to support the health of your kidneys.

Chapter 15: Conclusion

By the time you finish reading "The Renal Diet Meal Prep for the Newly Diagnosed: Delicious Low-Sodium Potassium Recipes to Manage Kidney Disease," you should take some time to evaluate the path you've taken and the positive effects of living a renal-friendly lifestyle. Building long-term kidney health habits and empowering yourself with a renal-friendly lifestyle are the main topics of this final chapter.

15.1 Empowering Yourself with a Renal-Friendly Lifestyle

Although being diagnosed with kidney disease can seem intimidating at first, adopting a renal-friendly lifestyle is a proactive and powerful step in taking control of your health. In terms of renal health, empowerment entails the following essential components:

1. Knowledge is Power

Gaining understanding about renal disease, its complexities, the value of a renal diet, and the significance of meal preparation will enable you to make well-informed decisions regarding your health. You have studied the intricacies of kidney health, investigated the fundamentals of a renal diet, and acquired useful knowledge about meal planning for ideal kidney function throughout this eBook.

- **Continued Learning:** Continue to be interested and inquisitive about kidney health. New discoveries and research advancements might provide further understanding that will strengthen your path.
- **Stay Informed:** Check reputable sources frequently for information on dietary guidelines, lifestyle choices that promote your wellbeing, and kidney health updates.

2. Taking Control of Your Diet

Making the right food choices is essential to managing renal illness. You may take control of what goes into your meals and make sure they follow renal-friendly rules by actively engaging in meal preparation.

- **Meal Planning Mastery:** Make the most of the information in this eBook to plan and cook meals that suit your tastes and lifestyle while also promoting renal health.

- **Cooking with creativity:** Try out new flavors, try renal-friendly dishes, and find inventive methods to prepare wholesome yet tasty meals.

- **Empowering Food Choices**: Choose foods that will improve your health. Choose foods that are high in nutrients and good for your kidneys, and pay attention to serving quantities.

3. Collaborating with Your Healthcare Team

A great helper in your path to renal health is your healthcare team, engaging in active collaboration with them guarantees that your strategy is tailored, knowledgeable, and compliant with the most recent medical advice.

- **Open Communication:** Encourage a culture of open communication with your nutritionist, nephrologist, and other medical professionals. Ask questions, voice your concerns, and participate actively in conversations about your health.

- **Regular Check-ups:** Follow your healthcare team's recommendations for routine check-ups and screenings. These consultations offer chances for treatment plan adjustments, monitoring, and the discussion of new health concerns.

4. Lifestyle Adaptations

Kidney health is influenced by a number of lifestyle factors in addition to nutrition. Make deliberate decisions that enhance your general well-being to empower yourself.

- **Physical Activity:** Include regular, kidney-friendly exercise in your daily routine. Keeping active improves your general health, whether you choose to walk, swim, or do little exercise.
- **Stress Management:** Practice stress-reduction strategies like mindfulness, meditation, or deep breathing exercises. Stress management improves renal health as well as mental wellbeing.
- **Adequate Sleep:** Since good sleep is so important to general health, make it a priority. Establish a sleep-friendly environment and cultivate good sleeping habits.

5. Advocating for Your Well-being

Speaking up for your wellbeing as the steward of your health is a powerful move. Take an active role in choosing your lifestyle and level of care.

- **Ask Questions:** If there is anything unclear regarding your treatment plan, nutritional advice, or kidney health, get clarification and ask questions.

- **Second Opinions:** To make sure you fully understand your options in complex situations or while making important decisions, don't be afraid to get second opinions.

- **Expressing Preferences:** Let your medical team know about your objectives and preferences. Collaborating with others guarantees that your treatment plan is in line with your values and way of life.

15.2 Building Long-Term Habits for Kidney Health

Achieving renal health is a marathon, not a sprint, developing enduring habits guarantees that you will always put your kidneys and general health first in your old age.

1. Consistency in Meal Preparation

Meal preparation is a habit that you can incorporate into your everyday life rather than just a temporary solution. Meal prep consistency guarantees that you make kidney-friendly decisions every time.

- **Weekly Meal Planning:** Keep up your weekly schedule for meal preparation. Set aside time to prepare ingredients, make shopping lists, and plan your meals for the following week.

- **Variety and Enjoyment:** Mix up your meals to keep your renal diet interesting. Taste new foods, experiment with recipes, and rejoice when you find exquisite flavors that are good for your kidneys.

2. Mindful Eating Practices

Eating with awareness is a practice that goes beyond a renal diet. It makes eating a joyful experience and promotes general wellbeing.

- **Mindful Eating Practices:** During meals, practice cultivating present-moment awareness. To develop a closer relationship with your food, focus on its flavors, textures, and colors.

- **Appreciation for Nourishment:** Learn to be appreciative of the food that you eat. Recognize the work and attention to detail that goes into making kidney-friendly, health-promoting meals.

3. Regular Physical Activity

Engaging in physical activity is a lifetime habit that supports kidney health as well as general wellness. Creating a routine around your preferences can guarantee long-lasting effects.

- **Incorporate Enjoyable Activities:** Opt for physical pursuits that fulfill and cheer you up. Make fitness a joyful aspect of your life, whether it is through dancing, gardening, or your favorite sport.

- **Consistency over Intensity:** Give consistency a higher priority than intensity. In the long term, regular, moderate exercise is more helpful and durable than intensive, irregular workouts.

4. Ongoing Self-Reflection

Sustaining kidney health requires ongoing introspection. Examine your habits on a regular basis, adapt as necessary, and acknowledge your accomplishments.

- **Journaling:** If you want to record your journey, think about keeping a journal. Jot down your feelings, ideas, and observations about your general well-being, lifestyle modifications, and renal diet.

- **Goal Setting:** Establish attainable, reasonable goals for the health of your kidneys. Review and modify these objectives on a regular basis in light of your development and changing priorities.

5. Seeking Support

Creating enduring habits requires teamwork. Seek for assistance from loved ones, groups, and friends who have similar health objectives.

- **Connect with Others:** Be a part of online communities or support groups where people with kidney illness exchange advice, encouragement, and experiences. Creating a network of support may be a source of inspiration and unity.
- **Involvement of Family and Friends:** Include your immediate family in your health journey. In order to create an atmosphere of understanding and support, let them know about your objectives, preferences, and difficulties.

6. Lifelong Learning

Continue to participate in lifelong learning. Your growing knowledge of kidney health may be influenced by fresh perspectives, scientific discoveries, and developments in the medical field.

- **Stay Informed:** Make sure you are aware of any changes in renal diets, lifestyle choices, and kidney health. To increase your expertise, go to conferences, webinars, and courses that are pertinent.

- **Adaptability to Change**: Have the willingness to modify your routines and habits as necessary. Adopt a growth mentality and acknowledge that new knowledge and experiences may cause your strategy to change.

You've started a journey toward empowerment and long-term wellness as you close this eBook. You've made great progress in properly managing kidney illness by learning about the subtleties of kidney health, adopting a renal-friendly lifestyle, and developing enduring habits.

Keep in mind that every person's journey is different, and achieving kidney health may involve both obstacles and successes. Appreciate your accomplishments, get help when you need it, and never waver in your commitment to your general health and kidney health.

Your commitment to living a renal-friendly lifestyle is an investment in your health now and in the future. Know that you have the resources, know-how, and fortitude to get through this path effectively; regardless of how long you've been an advocate for kidney health or how recently you received your diagnosis.

Carry with you the qualities of resilience, curiosity, and empowerment as you go. A fulfilling, kidney-healthy life is ahead thanks to your dedication to a renal-friendly lifestyle, which is a testament to your proactive attitude to health. I hope your journey is full of years of delicious, kidney-friendly foods, vibrant well-being, and ongoing empowerment.

About the Author

Dr. Adam C. stands as a beacon of inspiration in the fields of medicine, nutrition, and self-help, with a remarkable journey that exemplifies the transformative power of healthy living. Armed with a professional master's degree in health nutrition and years of experience, Dr. C. has become a guiding light for individuals seeking to embrace vibrant well-being and lead happier lives.

From an early age, Dr. C. navigated through a myriad of health challenges that ranged from genetic predispositions to the pitfalls of unhealthy eating. His personal struggle ignited a flame of determination within him, one that was fueled by the belief that the human body possesses an incredible ability to heal and rejuvenate through the right nourishment. Through steadfast dedication, Dr. C. managed to conquer his own ailments and emerged as a living testament to the transformative potential of a well-balanced lifestyle.

What sets Dr. Adam C. apart is his rich tapestry of experiences, having been deeply immersed in groundbreaking research in health food and diet-related domains. His quest to uncover the hidden treasures of nutrients within our meals has led to groundbreaking revel actions that empower individuals to extract the maximum benefit from their dietary choices. Dr. C.'s research has not only contributed to the scientific community but has also served as a roadmap for countless individuals striving to optimize their health.

However, it is not just Dr. C.'s academic prowess that has touched lives it is his unparalleled compassion and empathy that truly make him a beacon of hope. His personal journey of triumph over adversity infuses his guidance with an authentic understanding of the challenges his readers and patients face. Dr. C. doesn't just prescribe nutritional plans; he fosters a deep connection with his audience, instilling in them the confidence to embark on their own transformative journeys.

Dr. Adam C.'s holistic approach reaches beyond the confines of traditional medicine. His insights have translated into self-help resources that empower individuals to take charge of their wellness narrative. His words resonate on paper as they do in person, making his books not mere guides, but trusted companions on the path to vitality.

In the realm of health and nutrition, Dr. C. shines as a true luminary. His core strengths lie in his ability to synthesize complex scientific findings into practical, actionable advice that individuals from all walks of life can seamlessly integrate into their routines. Dr. C.'s legacy is not just a collection of breakthroughs; it is a testament to the extraordinary potential that lies within each of us to overcome obstacles and embrace a life brimming with health, happiness, and fulfillment.

As an experienced doctor, passionate nutritionist, and empathetic author, Dr. Adam C. continues to transform lives, showing us that the journey to a healthier, happier existence is within our grasp, waiting to be unlocked through the power of informed choices and unwavering determination.